EXPLORATIONS IN ETHICS

EXPLORATIONS IN ETHICS

READINGS FROM ACROSS THE CURRICULUM

Philip A. Rolnick
Editor

Rebecca F. Blomgren
Judy Cheatham
Nancy M. McElveen
W. Barnes Tatum
Associate Editors

Thomas A. Langford
Charles S. McCoy
Jeffrey Wattles
External Editors

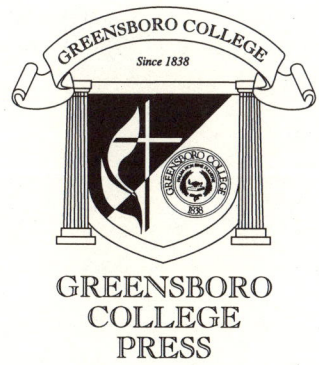

GREENSBORO
COLLEGE
PRESS

EXPLORATIONS IN ETHICS
READINGS FROM ACROSS THE CURRICULUM

Philip A. Rolnick
editor

Copyright © 1998 by Greensboro College Press

All rights reserved. No part of this work may be reproduced or transmitted in any form or by any means, electronic or mechanical, including photocopying and recording, or by means of any information storage or retrieval system, except as may be expressly permitted by the 1976 Copyright Act or in writing from the publisher.

Library of Congress catalog number 98-74049
ISBN 0-9667374-0-7

Printed in the United States of America
on acid-free paper

THIS BOOK IS DEDICATED TO

JANE AND ROYCE REYNOLDS

FRIENDS AND BENEFACTORS
OF
GREENSBORO COLLEGE

TABLE OF CONTENTS

Introduction
    Philip A. Rolnick .... *ix*

Foreword I: Ethics Across the Curriculum
    Daniel N. Keck .... *xi*

Foreword II: Ethics Across the Community and
New Generations
    Craven E. Williams .... *xvii*

INTRODUCTORY ARTICLE

What is Ethics?
    Philip A. Rolnick 3

PART ONE: CHRISTIAN ETHICS

Love as the Foundational Category for a Christian Ethic:
From Command to Virtue
    W. Barnes Tatum 27

Ethics in Methodism
    Thomas A. Langford 47

The Golden Rule Across the Curriculum
    Jeffrey Wattles 59

Christian Ethics: Jesus Christ, Covenant and Creation
    Charles S. McCoy 71

PART TWO: ACROSS THE CURRICULUM

This Is My Job: Freshman English in a Postmodern Age
   George Cheatham *95*

The Value of Literature in an Ethics Across the Curriculum Program
   of a Liberal Arts College
   Charles Hebert *121*

What Matters for Good Government?
   Nancy M. McElveen *131*

Ethics in History: A French Conscience
   Richard Francis Crane *155*

Ancient Wisdom for Educators and Parents: Proverbial Wisdom from Socrates,
   the Old Testament and Confucius
   John Hemphill *169*

Attending Beauty: The Inherent Ethic of Participation in Art
   Ray Martin *193*

Game Theory, the Classical Microeconomic Paradigm,
   and the Economics of Ethics
   Frederick J. Oerther, III *201*

Killing and Allowing to Die
   L. Alan Sasser *215*

Contributors *229*

INTRODUCTION

Explorations in Ethics: Readings from Across the Curriculum represents the current evolution of Greensboro College's Ethics Across the Curriculum (EAC) Program and the individual evolution of the faculty and distinguished guest speakers whose articles are included in this book. "Across the Curriculum" is an account by Vice President for Academic Affairs Daniel Keck of how and why the ethics program was begun at Greensboro College. "Across the Community" is an account by President Craven Williams of how and why the ethics program has been extended into the public schools of our area.

The text itself is a collection of articles in a number of disciplines written by Greensboro College faculty and three scholars from other institutions who have been guest speakers at Greensboro College. These articles represent a broad range of views and interests. The text, considered as a whole, represents a sort of composite snapshot of a moving reality. Yet, as is often the case in anthologies, the entire text may be adopted for classroom use, or alternatively, particular articles or areas may be used.

Explorations in Ethics begins with an introductory article that asks, "What Is Ethics?" This article explores the very nature of ethics and how raising the question of ethics leads to larger questions about the meaning of human life, especially our understanding of God in a global and diverse community.

Part One, "Christian Ethics," includes four articles. In the first, love is examined in the writings of representative Roman Catholic and Protestant theological ethicists. The article then follows the trajectory of love as it has been understood through the centuries of biblical redaction and concludes with contemporary documents of the United Methodist Church and the United Nations. While also referring to social creeds of the Methodist Church, the second article focuses on the historical development of ethics in the Methodist tradition, from John Wesley through influential writers of the present. The third article is a reflection on the golden rule. The last article in this section offers an overview of Christian ethics based on "Jesus Christ, Covenant, and Creation."

Part Two, "Across the Curriculum," includes eight articles by members of the Greensboro College community. The first two articles, by English professors, variously engage the issue of "canon" in teaching literature to undergraduates. The first argues for an intertextual approach while the second argues that some generally recognized canon would be worth retaining. The third article, written by a professor of French, discusses "What Matters for Good Government" in Plato's *Republic*, in the writings of *moralistes* of the sixteenth and seventeenth centuries, such as Fénelon, Bossuet, and Montesquieu, and in our own times. The fourth, written by a history professor, asks about the ethics of historical memory as it presents a case study in courage, the resistance of General Louis Eugène Faucher to the appeasement of Hitler at Munich and his later arrest by the Nazis. The fifth article, written by an education professor, examines wisdom in Socrates, the Hebrew Book of Proverbs, and Confucius. The sixth, reflecting the thinking of an art professor (who also contributes the cover design to this volume), argues that active participation in beauty can reveal a holistic vision of human life, one that ultimately leads to love. The seventh, by an economist, examines the criticisms of the Classical Microeconomic Paradigm (CMP), how the relatively recent development of Game Theory, when combined with the CMP, can overcome the criticisms against free market theory that are at the heart of the CMP, and how Game Theory even implies an economic basis for ethics. Finally, the book concludes with an examination of physician-assisted suicide. Its author, a former pastor, hospital chaplain, and consultant in these matters, describes the current state of the question and presents his own views of what should and should not be done.

Each of the individual articles is followed by questions for further discussion, generated by an education professor, that identify and probe themes addressed in the texts. The questions are provided with the hope of engendering classroom and other group discussions of these issues in ethics.

While there are many anthologies of ethics, this book is distinctive in that its subject matter arises out of one college's cooperative effort to approach ethics "across the curriculum." All the contributors have been participants in Greensboro College's Ethics Across the Curriculum Program, either as members of ongoing research symposia or as visiting lecturers. Furthermore, the editorial board, which has been actively involved in critiquing each of the articles included in this volume, represents four different teaching areas. While the diversity of viewpoints has at times made editorial consensus harder to achieve, we hope that the resulting product, *Explorations in Ethics* speaks in a more balanced way and to more diverse interests.

Philip A. Rolnick
Greensboro, August 1998

ETHICS ACROSS THE CURRICULUM

Daniel N. Keck

This collection of essays represents an important milestone in the development of the Ethics Across the Curriculum program at Greensboro College. The Ethics Across the Curriculum concept was introduced initially in an address which I delivered at an Academic Convocation in January 1992, shortly after my appointment as Vice President for Academic Affairs and Dean of the Faculty. The address, entitled "Paths to Distinctiveness," was intended to begin a dialogue with the faculty about future directions for the academic program at Greensboro College.

Of the several program initiatives which I suggested in that address, the Ethics Across the Curriculum program was the one most directly connected with my experiences as a political scientist, a classroom instructor, a lecturer, and an observer of American democracy at work.

As a political scientist, I was and continue to be intrigued by the debate as to the role that ethical and moral considerations should play in the relations of nation-states in general and in the formulation of American foreign policy in particular. My undergraduate and graduate education took place at a time when the dominant school of thought among theorists of international politics was the realist school, which contended that international relations can best be described as a never-ending struggle for power. Hans Morgenthau and other advocates of this theory argued that statesmen must be guided by the values of the state whose interests they were sworn to protect and that universal moral principles were of little relevance as a guide to the exercise of power in the international realm.[1]

At the same time that I studied theories of international relations, I also studied the history of American foreign policy in which universal moral principles often were invoked as a basis for American policies and actions in the world arena. I began my teaching career at the height of the Vietnam War, when debates about the morality of American involvement in Southeast Asia took place not only in college and university classrooms but also occupied a central place in our national political discourse.

The term debate is somewhat of a misnomer in that there was little effort on either side to engage the other intellectually. Rather, the political rhetoric was emotionally charged and aimed at solidifying political support or garnering the support of the media. These exchanges seldom resulted in a clarification of issues and almost never in the identification of any common ground between the opposing camps. Two other observations were important in deepening my interest in the subject. First, ethical principles often were used as an afterthought to justify political positions rather than being the basis for the positions themselves. And, second, many of these debates took place on quite superficial levels, with poorly constructed arguments and an absence of intellectual consistency and integrity.

I became convinced that, if debates about the role of ethics in international politics and foreign policy were to become meaningful, citizens would have to become better informed, not just about the issues but about the subject of ethics itself. So, I began to give a higher priority to the discussion of the ethical dimensions of issues in my classes and attempted to foster a more sophisticated approach to the complexities of this study on the part of my students.

Both in my classes and in a series of public lectures, I argued that a major source of difficulty in having a meaningful dialogue about the ethics of a particular international political issue was the fact that the participants in the dialogue often approached the issue from quite different perspectives. Using American foreign policy toward the Arab-Israeli dispute as an example, I stated that it was possible to analyze the ethical dimensions of this issue either from the perspective of universal moral values (e.g., peace, justice, and self-determination), or from the perspective of the national values of the United States (e.g., security and access to critical natural resources). The perspective of a particular group within the United States sometimes provided a third approach. In this particular case, many American Jews had an ethical perspective influenced by their identification with the state of Israel.

This analysis was helpful to my audiences in explaining why participants in debates about the ethics of a given international issue often seemed to be talking past one another rather than to one another. But these lectures and the discussions which followed them also demonstrated that such an analysis left critical questions unanswered. For example, even if all participants in a debate agreed to focus on universal moral values, several problems still remained: What are the universal moral values? How are these values to be defined? What happens when two or more universal moral values come into conflict with one another?

Out of these questions came my understanding of the importance of having a clear moral reference point—an ethical "anchor"—which would at least provide a framework for discussing these questions. This conclusion was to have a significant impact some years later in the thinking that guided the development and implementation of the Ethics Across the Curriculum program.

When I left full-time teaching and began a career in academic administration, I quickly realized that the potential for educating students about the ethical dimensions of issues existed in virtually every discipline. Students in biology, for example, should understand the ethical implications and consequences of genetic engineering. Students in education should have to grapple with the ethical issues involved in decisions about educating the learning disabled. From this realization, the concept of Ethics Across the Curriculum began to take shape. The goal was to ensure that all graduates of Greensboro College would have a sensitivity to the ethical dimensions of issues related to the subjects they studied and the ability to formulate well-reasoned responses to these ethical questions.

In 1994, Dr. Craven E. Williams, President of the College, announced a major gift from Jane and Royce Reynolds to support the College's Chaplaincy and Campus Ministry Program and to establish an Ethics Across the Curriculum program at Greensboro College. In announcing this gift, Dr. Williams stated that the purpose of this program "is to address the ethical issues which arise in every business and profession. We are a College of the Church, our heritage is in the United Methodist Church, and we eagerly look forward to expanding our mission in higher education as an expression of the Church's commitment to education."

With funding assured, planning for the Ethics Across the Curriculum program began in earnest. In discussing appropriate faculty development activities, Dr. Philip A. Rolnick, who was named director of the program, noted that most of our faculty had had no formal training in the subject of ethics. Given that fact, Dr. Rolnick argued persuasively that the initial focus of the program should be on giving faculty participants a solid grounding in the subject itself. Following that, the focus could shift to applying ethical principles to issues in the various disciplines.

In our discussions, we also addressed another significant issue, that of moral relativism. My earlier difficulties in applying ethical principles to international political issues taught me the limitations of an approach which stated that all ethical systems have equal validity. Acceptance of that viewpoint would mean that Morgenthau was correct—that universal moral principles had little relevance to the world of international politics. There is, I think, an important difference between acknowledging the existence of different and conflicting ethical systems and the conclusion that one therefore cannot (or at least should not) make judgments about the merits of these systems. From our standpoint, the College's Statement of Mission provides clear guidance on this point: "Greensboro College, an independent, co-educational college affiliated with the United Methodist Church, is an academic and social community which unites the liberal arts and Judeo-Christian values in an atmosphere of diversity and mutual respect." While acknowledging and respecting other ethical systems, the ethical "anchor" for this program would be the values inherent in the Judeo-Christian tradition.

The Ethics Across the Curriculum program formally began in the summer of 1995 with two faculty seminars which attracted twenty-two participants. More than 40% of the faculty, representing fifteen separate disciplines, participated in these seminars. Faculty members read and discussed Plato's *Republic* and several other philosophical works. The following summer, faculty participants continued their general study of ethics and also began to focus on applications in the various disciplines. A number of the chapters in this volume are an outgrowth of these studies.

The Ethics Across the Curriculum program also has sponsored a lecture series, bringing noted speakers to campus to speak on ethical issues. Dr. Thomas A. Langford, Professor of Theology and Methodist Studies and former Dean of the Divinity School at Duke University, presented the inaugural lecture in this series, entitled "Ethics: In Search of Foundations." Other speakers have included Dr. Jean Bethke Elshtain, Professor of Social and Political Ethics at the University of Chicago; Dr. Gilbert Meilaender, Professor of Ethics and Theology at Oberlin College; Dr. Jeffrey Wattles, Associate Professor of Philosophy at Kent State University; and Dr. W. C. Turner, Associate Professor of Homiletics at the Duke University Divinity School.

Students at Greensboro College have been actively involved in planning campus-wide events which are a part of the Ethics Across the Curriculum program. Each year, a student ethics committee has selected a theme and then developed programs around that theme. During the 1996-97 academic year, the student committee sponsored four well-attended panel discussions on topics related to ethics in sport. In 1997-98, the student committee sponsored a two-part program on the topic of affirmative action, which featured Charles S. McCoy, Robert Gordon Sproul Professor Emeritus of Theological Ethics at Pacific School of Religion in Berkeley, in favor of affirmative action and Gordon Dean Booth, a prominent attorney, who argued against affirmative action.

Another important facet of the Ethics Across the Curriculum program has been a series of faculty symposia. Each month during the academic year, a group of faculty gathers for lunch or dinner and a presentation by a member of the Greensboro College faculty on a particular ethical issue. Following the presentations, participants have the opportunity to discuss the presentation and to debate issues raised. Both presenters and participants have represented a wide range of disciplines at the College. Support for the symposia among faculty has been enthusiastic.

The Ethics Across the Curriculum program has been complemented by the establishment of an academic minor in ethics, which is an integral part of the offerings of the Religion and Philosophy program. The ethics minor, available to all students regardless of major, provides the opportunity for an in-depth study of the subject.

The study of ethics also will be reflected in the general education requirements of the College. As part of its current review of the general education requirements, the faculty debated and unanimously adopted a set of objectives for our general education program. "To think critically about ethics and values" is one of six general objectives. Students initially will explore ethics from the Judeo-Christian perspective in required courses in Old Testament and New Testament. This objective also will be infused in other general education courses, when appropriate, as well as in courses in every major. The inclusion of this objective reflects the commitment of the faculty to the importance of educating our students about ethics.

The key elements of the Ethics Across the Curriculum program as described in this introduction will continue. A second group of faculty recently has begun the two-year faculty seminar designed to give participants a broader understanding of the topic of ethics in general as well as its application to their respective disciplines. Faculty symposia, public lectures, and student-initiated programs will continue in a concerted effort to reach as many members as possible of both the campus and greater Greensboro communities. A second volume of essays already is planned. The next new initiative will be the integration of the study of ethics and values into a broad range of general education courses. This will represent a significant milestone in the implementation of the Ethics Across the Curriculum program at Greensboro College.

NOTES

1. Hans J. Morgenthau, *Politics among Nations: The Struggle for Power and Peace*, 4th ed. (New York: Alfred A. Knopf, 1967), 9-14, 219-249.

ETHICS ACROSS THE COMMUNITY
NEW GENERATIONS

Craven E. Williams

One important extension of the Ethics Across the Curriculum program at Greensboro College has been the New Generations Conferences and the Character Education Council developing from them. On February 26, 1997, and then again on March 11, 1998, more than 300 students, parents, teachers, and civic leaders gathered at Greensboro College for New Generations Conferences. In these meetings, first high school students, then middle school students, talked candidly in small groups with adults about their opportunities and obstacles, their potential and their problems. These young people were both encouraged by the attentive audience and curious to see how the community would respond to the anxieties they expressed.

The New Generations Conferences were initiated by the ten Rotary Clubs of Guilford County. They turned to Greensboro College to lead this effort for the 60,000 students in 94 schools in the county system because the Greensboro College faculty had actively demonstrated a desire to make ethics a pervasive element of the College curriculum.

Listening to the various participants in the discussions across our campus, I became convinced that we have undertaken a most significant enterprise. There is great value in understanding cultural differences; but the ultimate good is served when our citizens—young and old—value and respect each other and work together to identify common cornerstones of character, including an understanding of those components of character necessary for individual, communal, and national success. And so discussions about character, the community, and the individual filled the halls of Greensboro College for these two days.

Once, such discussions were common in public education. From the time of the ancient Greeks, in fact, to some time in the late nineteenth century, most people shared the notion that the mission of education went beyond academic content to include the modeling of character. By precept and example, education sought to make women and men better people. Thus, through education individuals were to become not only better informed but also more capable of controlling their emotions and conduct. The hope was that the informed and knowledgeable person would have the self-esteem and self-control to stand confidently in the face of adversity.

This two-pronged approach to education, content and character, was the norm in the United States until the mid-1960s, when, for a variety of reasons, character components were eliminated from the discussions in public schools across the country. The teaching of character was relegated to the home or the faith community.

Unfortunately, the consequences of this displacement became readily apparent, as crime rates, drug use, teen pregnancies, and other problems have increasingly plagued America's young people. Of course, these problems have multiple and complex roots; they also have multiple and complex solutions. Happily, one such solution has been the inception of the New Generations Program, which is a return to the two-pronged approach to education: content *and* character.

These days, young people have so much to learn. In this century, Americans have seen the transformation from an agrarian to an industrial society. Change has come from the mobility provided by cars and airplanes and now spaceships. Our television and fast food generation has gone from dancing the shag to discovering the stock market; we have survived Elvis and Madonna, rock and roll and rap. Boomers have gone from Vietnam to Bosnia, from the typewriter to hypertext. Now, a younger generation must cope in warpspeed with the mindboggling forces shaping today's society. In fact, the life that awaits them requires readiness for the changing dynamics of the family, for careers that do not yet exist, for a future we can barely imagine.

As we prepare young people for the twenty-first century, it is only fitting and natural to think about what is truly important, about what really matters. When everything is changing around us, does anything stay the same? If certain skills, occupations, and social structures become obsolete, are there any cornerstones, any constants? I contend that character is the constant. But what constitutes character? And who is truly qualified to teach it? If character is the key and the constant in our lives, we must define our terms, because whether we know it or not, we all teach character through the way we live our lives.

To begin, goodness has everything to do with character—not perfection or sainthood, not the impossible, but hardworking, trying your best goodness; making mistakes and admitting them and trying to fix them goodness; day in and day out goodness. The goodness of action. The ancient and universal axiom, "Do unto others as you would have them do unto you," begins with a verb of action.

In the goodness of action, growing out of the New Generations Conferences, a Character Education Council has been formed. The membership represents the diverse socio-economic, ethnic and faith communities of Guilford County. Citizens from all walks of life are working together in the difficult and challenging formative stages of this venture.

Certainly, the individual, with responsibility for self, develops his or her character. But there is also collective character, the character of the society as a whole, with responsibility to and for others. Social science calls this "collective efficacy." In fact, some studies show that a predictor of lower rates of violent crime is collective efficacy, the presence of a sense of trust, of common values and cohesion in neighborhoods. Furthermore, the important characteristic of collective efficacy is the willingness by residents to intervene in the lives of their children. This sense of community does not seem to depend on strong personal or kinship ties, as in a traditional village. Rather, it depends on a shared vision, a sense of engagement and ownership of public space.

In the goodness of action, the Character Education Council has developed a mission statement: to promote ethical standards to all Guilford County students as an integral part of their school training. Working with material generated by the students themselves, the Character Education Council is focusing on character traits commonly valued in all faith communities and ethnic groups: respect, compassion, responsibility, courage, integrity, perseverance, self-discipline, and generosity. Surely, with these traits as cornerstones, our community can move toward commonly shared positions.

In these ancient and honorable concepts, the youth of Guilford County have articulated their dreams for the new century. Like Martin Luther King, Jr., they have put the emphasis on the content of character, not on possessions, social position, class, or race.

Character acting in and through community is the focus of New Generations. The program extends the work of the smaller community, Greensboro College, and takes it into the larger community, Guilford County. In the twenty-first century, we can not be so parochial as to teach only the content; we must also teach the character. I contend that our future depends upon it.

INTRODUCTORY ARTICLE

WHAT IS ETHICS?

Philip A. Rolnick

ABSTRACT

Asking about ethics leads us, as it led Aristotle, to ask about the very meaning of human life. We cannot really say what the Good is or what we ought to do until we have answered the most basic questions of life itself, especially the question about God. The existence (or nonexistence) of God as well as how we understand God inevitably affect the way that we understand ourselves, our communities, and what we think human life ought to be like. The failure to believe in something that transcends our own point of view leads to ethical skepticism, which in turn tends to reduce human endeavor to the attainment of power. On the other hand, the very possibility of education implies that there is a transcendent goal to which we should aspire. In the ever-increasing diversity of our current global culture, understandings of God and humankind are necessary that are global in their inclusiveness. Love, as revealed in Jesus' teachings, should be our ultimate virtue and the goal of ethics.

Ethics begins in freedom and consistently displays the wild card of human choice. In its turn, human choice displays the somewhat more predictable *tendencies* of an underlying character. The dynamic interplay of choice and character is never an isolated, individual occurrence; rather, this interplay takes place on the testing ground of human life in community, the ethical arena in which individual and community character is revealed.

Upon this testing ground ethics can be further understood as the sacred art of judgment. While numerous components enter into ethical reflection and behavior, such as thought, emotion, and prior tendencies, these components have an interplay that is synthesized in the act of judgment. In the countless activities of our lives, we are constantly evaluating options, assessing situations, and valuing one thing over another. What kind of value judgments we tend to make is always revealing of character. Thus judgment becomes one of our distinctively human activities. Animals may largely function on the level of instinct, and God may function on the level of perfection in all things, but human beings must function in a middle way, where the quality of judgment determines much of life, perhaps even destiny, as judgment culminates in action.

Much of the process that leads to judgment and action is inner and invisible. Within a human being is an array of possibilities—animal urges, passion and preference, vanity and honor seeking, thought, and perhaps even prayer, meditation, and worship. But once the interior process culminates in judgment leading to action, the publicness of ethics is manifest. In the public arena, actions and the judgments which lead to actions inevitably affect others in the community. Thus Aristotle considered ethics "in a sense an investigation of social and political matters";[1] in fact, from the Greek term for city (*polis*) we take our English term, "politics." Many Americans claim that they are "not political," and in the sense of seeking elected office or even knowing very much about the daily doings of government, they are probably right. But if we use the term more as Aristotle did, then we can redefine politics as "ethical reflection and interaction in a community." Then we can more easily recognize how political and ethical matters intertwine, how individual and community are mutually interactive. All human groupings, from the nuclear family to the entire global community, involve us in varying degrees and intensities of ethical interaction.

The inevitable, interactive, interpersonal aspect of ethical judgment leading to action means that what we say and do affects those around us. Hence, others have a stake in our ethical process. Ethics is never merely a "me, myself, and I" business. Human beings do not live in total isolation.

The fact that our behavior affects others and the equally important fact that others' behavior affects us throw us all into the ethical arena. There are no neutral positions and no omniscient referees to whom we have immediate access. Although countless people may attempt it, ethical "hiding" is impossible; for hiding itself becomes an ethical choice. Choosing not to think about how we affect others is still a choice, a choice by default. It just means that we would affect others unthinkingly, unintelligently. Ethical drift may accurately describe what many do, but once the ethical question has been acknowledged, it is possible to develop an ethical sense of direction.

ARISTOTLE'S QUESTION AND RESPONSE
SEEKING THE GOOD

Philosophical and religious traditions have in one way or another asked what human life should be. As Aristotle begins his classical study, the *Nicomachean Ethics*, he notes that we do many things for the sake of something else. But if we could determine an "end" or a purpose (*telos*) that we do strictly for its own sake, "then obviously this end will be the good, that is, the highest good. Will not knowledge of this good, consequently, be very important to our lives?"[2] In his elegant simplicity, Aristotle has already parsed much of the problem. So much of what we do, we do not for its own sake, but for the sake of some other perceived need or pleasure. Hence, many modern people (and the ancients were not all that different) spend the majority of their waking hours at jobs that they dislike in order to pay for things that they do like, such as cars, nice houses and clothes. The people caught up in this unthinking drift through life become the slaves of their possessions and processes unless they stop the process long enough to ask something like Aristotle's question and the ones that naturally follow from it: What is the highest good? and, How can I go about pursuing it in my life? Asking such questions bestows focus, serious movement, and perhaps an ethical sense of direction to our lives. If we could answer these questions, says Aristotle, "Would it not better equip us, like archers who have a target to aim at, to hit the proper mark?"[3] Once this question is asked, transcendence has begun. Now human intelligence is no longer limited to achieving things and pursuing creature comforts; human intelligence is now enlisted in asking about the purpose, the end, the *telos*, the big picture of our lives.

A question honestly asked has a way of leading to other questions. Aristotle, for instance, notes that flutists, sculptors, and carpenters all have well-defined functions. We know what they are supposed to do. But what is the function of human life itself? He rules out "simply living," since even plants do that. Surely, he muses, it cannot be the case that the parts have meaning, but there is none available to the whole.[4] And so, his question becomes: What does it mean to be human? And then moves on to ask what an *excellent* ("virtue" and "excellence" are equally good translations of Aristotle's term, *aretē*) human life would be like.

What would an excellent human life be like? We can begin to answer the question by specifying positive qualities of living that would make up the ethical life. In other words, we have already advanced beyond the popular notion that ethics is about not doing something, e.g., not stealing, not lying, not deliberately hurting others. These negative commands, like those found in the Ten Commandments, are not wrong. They have their necessary place in the ethical life. Freedom from bad habits may be a prerequisite to achieving good habits. In this sense avoiding the bad could be called pre-ethical behavior. Such avoidance is necessary but, in and of itself, insufficient. Teaching a young child not to put her hand on a hot stove is necessary for the child to learn, but a child needs to be taught more than what *not* to do. Avoiding the bad is not on the same level as doing the good. An excellent life must be based on the Good, and seeking the Good underlies all of classical ethics.

For Aristotle, seeking the Good and progressively achieving it is the route to excellence and the fulfillment of our humanity.[5] Each of us is born with a first nature, what we call heredity. Assuming that this first nature is reasonably sufficient, we can then develop, with the help of parents, teachers, and, we hope, the larger community, a second nature, what we would call character. In Aristotle's mind, children cannot possess virtue. They are potentially virtuous. The point of teaching and training children in the Good is to actualize their undeveloped potential. The process of actualizing potential becomes the goal of instruction and training. At its simplest, Aristotle's ethical program advocates actualization of potential through habituation in the Good.

Aristotle, working prior to the Christian tradition and apart from the Jewish tradition, is concerned about permanence and reliability. He knows that ethics must be more than just one or two good decisions or gracious responses. His movement toward character-based ethics seeks as much permanence and reliability as was possible in strictly human terms.[6] Noticing that things in nature possess permanent tendencies, Aristotle wants the virtuous human to have as much of the Good as possible and to have it as permanently as possible by practicing habits that are good and that promote the Good. He wants the habit of the Good to become so strong that it becomes second nature, and so the permanent possession of an excellent character. Nonetheless, as character is developed to the point of becoming second nature, the intellect remains active and alert. Habit does not imply automatic pilot.

While the lists of virtues vary, as do the preferred translations, four classical or "cardinal" virtues are generally recognized among the ancient Greeks: practical wisdom, self-control, courage, and justice or righteousness. These four, which are ingredients of the Good, are to be unified within the character of the excellent, virtuous human being.[7]

For Aristotle, character is never formed in a vacuum. Instead, there is a back and forth interaction, what modern ethicists call a dialectic, between the inner processes of an individual and the public nature of actions taken as a result of those inner processes. The interior and the exterior are closely related and intertwined. What we do affects who we are; what we are affects what we do. This has often been referred to as the "being/doing" dialectic. This dialectic is not static; it does not leave either component, who we are or what we do, as it was. Instead, what we are and what we do are both changed, hopefully improved, by ongoing interaction. Improvement will result if a good first nature is being given good instruction and training en route to a good second nature. All of Aristotle's program assumes that there is someone present—a parent, teacher, or perhaps the whole community—who knows at least something of the Good and is willing to work to inculcate it in the young.

QUESTIONING HUMAN HORIZONS

Human life is intensively lived among other human beings, so relations with others naturally take center stage in most of our ethical discussions. However, people clearly interact with more than just other people. What we do affects not only plant and animal life, but also the planetary, and, to a degree, the astronomical environment. Asking what it means to be human, asking what we ought to do in our lives, almost naturally leads the inquirer to the next question: What is the source of humanity? Does humanity have a destiny beyond what it creates for itself? And these questions provoke an ultimate question, the question about the source, purpose, and destiny of all reality: the question about God. How does God's existence, and our understanding of the divine existence, affect our understanding of what human life should be?

How one answers this question fundamentally shapes one's ethical possibilities—and hence one's humanity. Here again ethical (as well as theological) hiding is impossible. Problem avoidance works no better on this level than on any other known to us. Our most basic understandings of reality cannot help but shape our ethical perspective. How we answer the question about God frames our concept of humanity.

THE SOURCE OF ETHICAL SKEPTICISM

Answered negatively, atheistically, "man" then tends to become "the measure of all things."[8] Advocates of this sort of godlessness do not and cannot answer the question about the source of reality, and the question about destiny becomes rather meaningless. For them, the universe just is—a sort of fortuitous (for us), but nonetheless unplanned, happening. Once this position is adopted, ethics can only be, and ought to be, a purely human construction. Talk about God or a Supreme Being comes under the suspicion of glorifying and legitimizing the ethical directives of one's own tribe, race, or nation.[9] In this understanding, God becomes merely a fiction used to reinforce and empower human rules, regulations, and preferences. Given the assumptions of this way of perceiving the world, there is nothing outside or beyond humanity toward which we should aim. As a result, for advocates of this atheistic position, humankind is free to construct its own best versions of what is right. Since such positions tend toward ethical skepticism, i.e., they really suspect that there is no objective moral truth, ethics gives way to power. In Book I of Plato's *Republic*, Thrasymachus contends against Socrates that "justice is nothing other than the advantage of the stronger" (338c). In other words, whoever is in power determines what is just. Independently of those making the rules, there is no such thing as justice. Books II-IX of *The Republic* are Plato's attempt to defend justice and ultimately the Good, upon which justice rests.

In more modern times, the German philosopher Friedrich Nietzsche has advocated a similar position, characterizing Judeo-Christian morality as "slave morality" and Christianity as "the most fatal and seductive lie that has ever yet existed—as the greatest and most *impious* lie" ever practiced upon the human race.[10] Nietzsche, much like Thrasymachus, advocates that the strong should be unrestrained by the artificial constructs, the pious frauds, of the weak, especially Christianity. Instead, he wants to reach, as in the title of one of his works, "beyond good and evil" to the formation of the *Übermensch* (superman). It is no accident that, in both the ancient case of Thrasymachus and in the modern case of Nietzsche, once goodness is abandoned as something real, power takes over.

In John Milton's *Paradise Lost*, Satan and his followers are thrown from heaven after they rebel against the authority of God's Son. As they collect themselves amid the ugliness of the Hell in which they find themselves, Satan rallies his forces with the lure of power: "Better to rule in hell than serve in heav'n."[11] But is it better to rule in Hell? Is power and its distribution what is most basic to life? Is power all that there is?

To the ethical skeptic, power, winning, and looking good are demonstrable and real. From this point of view, one does not defend a position because it is true, or good, or right; one defends it because it is one's own. When one gives up a position, one gives up power and prestige. Philosophical, religious, and political differences are merely contests of force that pretend to be something else. Conversation under these conditions is not a means of sharing or learning but of defending one's own turf and attacking that of the other party, who can only be seen as the opponent and, more likely, the enemy.

There has always been a chasm of understanding between the skeptic and those who believe in something beyond themselves, something transcendent. The chasm is tellingly revealed in the biblical accounts of the trial of Jesus. When Jesus is brought before Pontius Pilate, the Roman governor and most politically powerful man in Jerusalem, Pilate does not ask Jesus about his teaching or his religion. He asks him about his power: "Are you the king of the Jews?" As the Gospel of John reports the conversation, after some discussion about what it means to be a king, Jesus moves the discussion to considerations of *truth*:

> For this I was born, and for this I have come into the world, to bear witness to the truth. Every one who is of the truth hears my voice. (John 18:37b-38)

Pilate's worldly reply, "What is truth?" is delivered from his position of power and reveals a jaded lack of interest in Jesus' topic. His answer displays once again the basic mindset of the skeptic: truth does not exist, and, if it does, we cannot know what it is. Across a chasm from Pilate stands Jesus, who, though on trial for his life, remains solely concerned with his mission of teaching truth. Pilate does not hear Jesus' voice. Instead, though he acknowledges Jesus' innocence, he finds it expedient to have Jesus scourged and crucified. As the biblical accounts variously portray this trial, judgment, and execution, Pilate consistently behaves in a manner that he thinks will protect his power with little or no concern for justice. To the skeptic, justice, like truth or goodness, is at best shadowy or, more likely, unreal. But those who prefer peace to war, those who prefer binding a wound to causing one, should think twice before advocating positions of ethical skepticism.

COMMUNITY, *WELTANSCHAUUNG*, AND INDIVIDUAL RESPONSE

Charles McCoy has pointed out that each of us wakes up in a world well underway before our arrival on the scene. We are introduced to reality through the interpretive filters of parents and relatives, teachers and ministers, and perhaps others:

> We receive and respond to patterns existing before our appearance. Gradually we are inducted into this community of interpretation, take our place within its relationships and interactions, and participate in revising its interpretations and passing them to subsequent arrivals.[12]

As newborns, we are sufficiently fragile that, without people going to a great deal of bother about each one of us, we would have no hope of negotiating our way into and through the complexities of human life. So, as McCoy points out, we are gradually inducted into responsibilities and relationships. Eventually, however, it becomes our responsibility to pass on to new arrivals what we have learned and perhaps discovered on our own, even if what we have discovered is in some ways challenging to previous teachings.

Michael Polanyi has called this process "Dwelling In and Breaking Out."[13] We all begin by receiving the nurture and instruction of the tradition(s) into which we are born. However, the creative individual often "breaks out" of traditional understandings on the way toward greater truth, which Polanyi defines as "the achievement of a contact with reality."[14] Each new "contact with reality," whether in science, philosophy, or religion, tends to unsettle or disrupt the equilibrium of the current community. However, each such contact with reality, each new furtherance of truth, is worth the disturbance; for it makes the community more *realistic*. That is, the tradition adapts, adjusts, or perhaps even changes its *Weltanschauung* to conform to the new discovery or revelation. In such cases, the change is a good change. It is creative and constitutes progress by advancing the community's hold on the true, the good, or the beautiful. However, without an objective, transcendent goal at which to aim, we could never evaluate whether a given change was good or bad. Change would become merely a matter of personal or community preference, and "progress" would become meaningless; for progress is only possible if a change advances our understanding of the reality of the physical world in science and the reality of the living God in religion. Hence Polanyi speaks of "contact with reality" and expresses the hope that we can "increase ever further our hold on reality."[15] "Contact with reality" gives seriousness and purpose to those who accomplish it and to those who accept the new developments. So, for example, the Copernican theory that the earth revolves around the sun arrives as an offensive shock to the European community of the 1500s, but once the more realistic theory is adopted, it eventually leads the later community to achieve space travel and, through satellite systems, vastly improved global communications networks on a previously unimaginable scale. The contact with reality enables us to do more. It makes us more powerful because it makes us more realistic.

Yet not all change is good. The destruction of community values, without replacing them with something greater, amounts to intellectual and spiritual vandalism. The shattering may be exciting and temporarily energetic, but it brings predictably negative consequences in its wake, as power becomes the only dependable reality. Those who dare to unsettle civilization must offer something better than what they would have us replace. Advocates of change bear the ethical responsibility to lead the larger community to something greater, not merely something different.

Different peoples and different individuals perceive the world differently. Our way of perceiving the world, our *Weltanschauung*, is not innocent. What we receive from others is already ethically charged. How we in turn transmit our *Weltanschauung* to others is our own ethical challenge. Telling another generation what the world is like is fraught with ethical weight. For example, in the Academy, as professors profess a position, as they emphasize some things and leave others aside, they are guiding the induction process. In creating a course syllabus, professors cannot escape making ethical judgments.

Unless the ethical skeptics are right, all ways of seeing the world are not born equal. Just as the blind do not physically see as well as those with 20/20 vision, neither do the foolish perceive what the wise see. As Plato suggests, the view of an expert navigator should not be equated with that of someone who has no experience at sea; likewise, the counsel of a scoundrel and that of a person of excellent character do not lead to the same results. The process of construing the world, which includes the best thinking that we can do, but also includes more than, not less than, rationality, constitutes much of the sacred art of judgment.

Even the language that we use is ethically charged. The very choice of the term "world," as opposed to "creation," is already ethically and theologically loaded. The real estate is the same, but the *Weltanschauung*[16], the way of perceiving it, differs greatly. Once we see the world and its greater universe as a creation, then we have already to some extent framed, focused, and begun to define our concept of humanity; for in a creation, there must be a Creator, a responsible source for the reality that we encounter in our lives and to whom we must ourselves be related. If, by right of birth, we are all related to the same Creator, then we must be related to one another. If the Creator is the responsible source for the reality in which we find ourselves, then responsibility, especially relational responsibility, is ingredient to humanity.

GIVENNESS, TRANSCENDENCE, AND HUMAN RESPONSE

To say that we exist because the Creator wanted to share life with us means that our lives are gifts. The New Testament term *charis* may be equally well translated as "gift" or "grace." Thomas A. Langford has argued that the entire tradition stemming from Wesley can be understood as "an extended consideration of the grace of God as expressed in Jesus Christ."[17] The Methodist tradition begins in the perception of the giftedness of our lives, but it goes further in seeking to stimulate an appropriate response of gratitude, especially as witnessed in service to others in the human family. Langford's emphasis on "*practical* divinity" (as in the title of his book) captures an important insight of the tradition—that in gratitude we should respond in practical ways to the gifts of Creation and Christ, to "grace upon grace" (John 1:16), gift upon gift. How God is understood shapes the ethical response.

Michael Novak, a Catholic writer, takes a point from John Locke (1632-1704) about intelligent human effort:

> Locke observed that a field of, say, strawberries, highly favored by nature, left to itself, might produce what seemed to be an abundance of strawberries. Subject to cultivation and care by practical intelligence, however, such a field might be made to produce not simply twice but tenfold as many strawberries. In short, Locke concluded, nature is far wealthier in possibility than human beings had ever drawn attention to before.[18]

Novak concludes from this and similar observations that the work of creation is unfinished—purposefully unfinished. Actualizing the potential found in creation bestows a sense of purpose on our humanity. In the transfer of competency from Creator to creature may be discovered something like the transfer of responsibility that takes place as human parents guide their children into full adulthood.

Seeing ourselves within the framework of Creation helps us perceive reality as planned and purposeful. In the sense that it would be absurd to say human beings invented strawberries, so too all human creativity is more akin to *discovery* than to raw invention or construction. Thus human beings are creative to the extent that we creatively conform to the patterns and principles of the Creation. We may not be able to invent strawberries, but we can and *ought to* discover ways of making them and countless other items of benefit broadly available. We can actively and intelligently cooperate with what God has already provided. Scientific endeavor is thus encouraged and positioned within the framework of appropriate human activities under God. Any development or increase of human power is thus related to a more transcendent power and purpose. Keeping the gifted nature of our existence before the mind has a salutary effect on human ego, which all too easily balloons to gigantic yet dangerously fragile proportions when we take ourselves as "the measure of all things."

The great Indian sage Gautama Siddhartha, when asked who he really was, denied that he was a god, an angel, or a saint. He replied simply: "I am awake." In fact, the title by which he would become known, the Buddha, means the "Awakened One."[19] Like the Buddha, we should be awake to the possibilities latent in the gift of life.

Transcendence and Education

Michael Polanyi contends that we must show a "preference for truth even at the expense of losing in force of argument. Nobody can practice this unless he believes that truth exists."[20] In comparing Polanyi's attitude to the Satan character in *Paradise Lost*, the ethical question, the question about life itself, strikes us with renewed force. Polanyi can say *"that truth exists."* On the other hand, the Satan of *Paradise Lost* will not say so. Instead, he prefers to win and to rule, even in Hell. Satan's preference makes perfectly good sense, "unless" we believe with Polanyi "that truth exists." Here, loyalty to truth counts more than any other contender for our loyalty. The *judgment* that Polanyi offers is that it is better to lose an argument if it means gaining the truth. For in gaining the truth, we could never really have lost anything. Instead, we have in some real sense bettered ourselves. Education has taken place.

In Plato's *Gorgias*, Socrates has angered a powerful young man named Callicles by refuting his argument. As Callicles refuses to continue the discussion, and as his anger rises to the level of actual threat to Socrates' well-being, Socrates offers this famous rejoinder:

> But since you are unwilling, Callicles, to help me finish the argument, you can at least listen and interrupt if at any point you think I am wrong. And if you refute me, I shall not be vexed with you as you are with me, but you shall be enrolled as the greatest of my benefactors. (*Gorgias* 506c)

Without the existence of truth, Socrates' speech makes no sense. Callicles could not become the greatest of Socrates' benefactors by *apparently* defeating him "unless [Socrates] believes that truth exists." But if truth does exist, no one could ever be defeated by being taught new truth. Yet without truth, education is unthinkable. No one could become a better person, or, for that matter, a worse one. Without truth, "better" and "worse" are demoted to mere preferences that individuals may have (or may not have). For Callicles, being weaker or stronger, more powerful or less so in social ranking, is what counts.

On the other hand, for those whose primary purpose is to seek the truth and the closely related good, conversation holds the promise of sharing good things, correcting wrong things, and eliminating bad things. Such is the reasoning of Socrates in Plato's Dialogues. What some modern bestsellers have called "win-win" is a retrieval and modern application of the wisdom already present in Plato.

Most important for us is that once we recognize something that transcends each one of us, whatever our position among our peers, power-seeking and the desire to look good may recede long enough for education to get underway. Education, which involves learning new things, is as much for teachers as for students. A teacher who has learned nothing new in the last decade holds the title rather tenuously. Socrates is unafraid of correction because he knows that it is the best possible thing that he could receive if wrong. Carrying wrong beliefs, wrong ideas, and wrong attitudes weighs us down on our journey and points us away from our real destination. It may even destroy us. The Thousand Year Reich, which began with such inebriated hopes (for its own people) ended ingloriously in just thirteen years, with millions of Germans (and millions of others) dead and Germany, the self-declared fount of power and mastery, an occupied country in rubble and ruin.

Education is not about coercive power. It has much more to do with humility. Paradoxically, humility has its own power—the power that can tap hidden resources because it is unafraid to undergo self-correction. Meekness, humility, is not weakness. Many of the most important figures in human history have been more characterized by humility than by conventional power. Consider that Moses, the liberator of the Hebrews, is described as, "very meek, more than all the men that were on the face of the earth" (Num. 12:3). Among others, the list might include Amos, Socrates, Jesus, Gandhi, Martin Luther King, Jr., and Mother Theresa. By not insisting on self-assertion, they reveal something which always manifests as fresh and new—a transcendent faith that challenges the rest of us to be more alert to our own possibilities—and to actualize them.

The educational enterprise has always involved listening, not just listening to other people, but listening to reality, whether understood on material, intellectual, or spiritual and personal levels. This kind of listening requires humility. The educational process is born in a dialectic between humility about one's own limitations and confidence in a transcendent reality that is to some degree accessible and discoverable under the right conditions of inquiry. No scientist would work endless hours trying to break new ground if he thought there was no new ground to break. No church or synagogue could long be maintained if people regarded God as only a projection of humankind. Believing that there is something beyond us is healthy for the human race. Without such belief, the educational enterprise could not be sustained, except perhaps by those schools that promoted and trained adherents in military strategy and other forms of power relations. But contests of power will be especially dangerous in the highly diverse context in which we now find ourselves.

TRANSCENDENCE AND PLURALISM

One of the most powerful movements of our time is the heightened awareness of diversity in human culture and belief. This heightened awareness has led, especially in American universities, to commitments to pluralism as part of a growing global awareness. In the proverbial phrase of Marshall McLuhan, the world is now a global village. Violence in any city of the globe can now appear on television screens throughout the world in a matter of minutes. Borders are increasingly permeable due to radio, television, fax machines, e-mail, the internet, and vastly more accessible and less expensive telephone networks. More people travel to more places than ever before imaginable. All in all, it is an exciting time to be alive.

As the United States in particular has attempted to incorporate waves of cultures, races, philosophies, and religions, our educational and religious institutions have had to adapt to the new conditions. While animosity, friction, and outright warfare among different groups is always a possibility and, in some nations, such as the former Yugoslavia, has become a reality, our civilization is not without the intellectual and spiritual tools to meet this latest ethical challenge.

The United States is in many ways a synthesis of two not always compatible, but variously lofty, ideals: the Reformation and the Enlightenment. The majority of Americans, albeit with a dazzling diversity of variations, count themselves among one of the Christian traditions. Yet the foundational political documents of the nation, the Declaration of Independence and the Constitution, are classic Enlightenment writings. In the Declaration we do not find theistic, christological, revelatory notions; instead, we find Deistic understandings consonant with the regnant Zeitgeist of natural law that was universally accessible through the exercise of reason, which was itself, like mathematics, assumed to be universally accessible to all people.

While English writers most directly affected the incipient political views of our nation, no Enlightenment figure has been more lastingly influential than Immanuel Kant. Kant's ethical views have often been summarized in his different statements of the Categorical Imperative:

> Act only according to that maxim by which you can at the same time will that it should become a universal law.
>
> Act so that you treat humanity, whether in your own person or in that of another, always as an end and never as a means only.[21]

Kant wants individuals to be autonomous, to make their own decisions in freedom about all aspects of their lives, including religion, ethics, politics, and medicine. Kant's purpose is not to promote anarchy through the overthrow of all authority. Rather, it is to promote enlightenment, the exercise of reason, and hence genuine morality by placing freedom and concomitant responsibility upon the individual. In the 1780s, Kant stands in the relatively early days of circumnavigation and expanded contact among the world's peoples and religions, and he sees trouble brewing. As authoritative religions and nation states collided, as they had in the Thirty Years War, additional warfare and strife could only be on its way. Against this worrisome backdrop of colliding cultures, nations, and religions, Kant has a vision of world peace based on laws of reason, which he contends are *universal* where authoritative religions are *particular* in an *exclusivistic* sense. Kant's universal vision, whether applied to the individual or to communities, is inseparable from his ethical commitment.[22] The individual has to be autonomous, free, so that universal responsibility can be exercised. Freedom is not the final end, just a necessary condition for the practice of genuine morality, which Kant understands as the exercise of universal responsibility.

Especially in his doctrine of universal respect for persons *as ends in themselves* does Kant offer something helpful to our current situation. When Kant speaks about a person being an "end in himself," he means that an individual human being is not fungible, not exchangeable. Individual dollar bills are fungible, but individual human beings are not because each individual is a unique personality. The value of each human being is already present in that *person*, apart from anything that person might have accomplished or contributed. While the full story is more complicated, Kant certainly has been influential in such later developments as the United Nations Declaration of Human Rights. In our pluralistic culture, something like Kant's respect for persons along with the practice of universal responsibility is now truly imperative.

EXCLUSIVISM AND UNIVERSALISM

The Judeo-Christian traditions that still shape so much of America's public and private understandings are not without new contributions to make in our time. The continuing influence of religion for good is sometimes hard to decipher, if only because there is such a plurality of religious voices. However, of the basic ethical divides in the religions of our time, the most important is that between religious exclusivism and universalism.

Exclusivism is more of a religious disposition than a trait which belongs to any one religion. It is found among Jews, Christians, Moslems, Sikhs, and others. The common idea is that God loves and favors "our" people and directs "us" to be separate from, to overcome, and even to destroy, if necessary, all others. Examples abound. In Deuteronomy, the Hebrews, who are about to enter the Promised Land, are directed:

> When the LORD your God brings you into the land which you are entering to take possession of it, and clears away many nations before you, the Hittites, the Girgashites, the Amorites, the Canaanites, the Perizzites, the Hivites, and the Jebusites, seven nations greater and mightier than yourselves, and when the LORD your God gives them over to you, and you defeat them; then you must utterly destroy them; you shall make no covenant with them, and show no mercy to them.... But thus shall you deal with them: you shall break down their altars, and dash in pieces their pillars, and hew down their Asherim, and burn their graven images with fire. (Deut. 7:1-5)

This passage demonstrates precisely the kind of religious exclusivism against which Kant and the Enlightenment generally did battle. Similarly, notions of Christian exclusivity, in which Christians are saved and others are the enemies of God, have at times been unleashed. The Crusades represent a historical example of Christian religious exclusivism. Rather a strange notion to kill infidels in the name of the Prince of Peace; yet, such is the embarrassing history. More recently, Islamic fundamentalists were responsible for the bombing of the World Trade Center in New York, killing several people, wounding many, and doing millions of dollars of damage. The men who performed that act of premeditated murder and destruction acted according to their best understanding of loyalty to their particularistic God.[23] The predictably violent and bitter fruits of religious exclusivism should be clear from these examples.

In our global village, religious exclusivism may serve its adherents well in some ways, but it fails almost any ethical test that we can devise. It fails the first statement of the Categorical Imperative because we cannot take the maxim of the action and make it a universal law. The world would fall into a permanent state of ethnic cleansing, crusade, or *jihad*. Religion itself would descend to the level of military power. Exclusivism fails the second statement of the Categorical Imperative because it utterly disrespects the personhood of the individuals who are murdered or maimed, as well as their families who are bereft. It even fails utilitarian considerations, since it can hardly produce the greatest good for the greatest number. Religiously motivated violence is far more likely to produce the opposite.

The best of Christian thinking joins hands with Enlightenment thinking in opposing dehumanization of other groups as blameworthy and in judging violence against outsider groups as despicable. The Catholic natural law tradition, which precedes Kant by many centuries, recognizes a unique value in each human being because we are, according to Gen. 1:26-27, made "in the image of God." Likewise, the practice of the golden rule, Do to others as you want others to do to you, has been championed in most of the major religions of the world.[24] The perpetrators of the World Trade Center bombing could hardly want their victims to do the same to them and to their families. Finally, Jesus of Nazareth, as he goes to his death on the Roman cross, neither threatens nor curses his executioners. Instead, he asks, "Father forgive them, for they know not what they do" (Luke 23:34). Religious understanding and commitments may often be so intertwined with ethical judgments that they are impossible to separate, even if one wanted to do so. How we understand the character of God has to shape the way that we would like our own character to be. Hence, a great deal is at stake in how we understand God.

It is not the case that the presence of many religions and ethical viewpoints means that we cannot or should not make judgments about particular claims. Such positions end up paralyzing the conversation. Just as Socrates is willing to be corrected by his conversation partners, religious encounters can become more and more meaningful through the ethic of listening, an ethic of humility. As we stand before the Transcendent, we could actually learn something from one another. The particular need not be exclusive. It can be a route toward the universal. As a Native American friend once put it, "There are many paths up the mountain."

While diversity is now a given, some movement toward oneness, toward common understanding and perhaps toward commonly held goals, would be an ethical achievement. Familiarity with other cultures and traditions is the latest development of planetary education in a global village. Adapting to new ideas is not a sign of weakness or disloyalty. It may be a movement to a greater understanding of reality. The founding fathers of the United States placed on the coinage of the realm "*e pluribus unum*" (out of the many, a one). These visionary forbears understood that even in that simpler time, they were already a diverse people, a people from many nations and religions. If a nation was going to be forged from the thirteen colonies that were so severely tested, then sufficiently universal principles had to be adopted in order to enlist the cooperation of the diverse people involved. Over the years, those principles have persistently needed to be broadened in their interpretation, such as in the achievement of the civil rights of African-Americans and in the voting rights of women. Just as the American narrative has a certain universalizing trajectory, so too does the global village now follow such a trajectory.

LOVE: THE ULTIMATE VIRTUE

Christianity is not without the resources to meet the demands of the changing times. Making sense of pluralism was part of the original strength of historic Christianity. Jews, Romans, Greeks, and others learned to cooperate, respect one another, and even love one another in the first decades after Jesus' life. While the institutional church has sometimes wandered into exclusivity, Jesus does not do so. The one who teaches the parable of the Good Samaritan, sometimes known as the parable of brotherly love (Luke 10:29-37), who permits women to accompany him on a preaching tour (Luke 8:1-3), something unheard of in that era, whose first reported resurrection appearances are to women, and who teaches the prayer which begins, "Our Father" (Matt. 6:9), should first of all be understood as aiming toward a universal, inclusive, and personal love which would culminate in a new realm: the global family of God. Indeed, Jesus goes so far as to command love of enemies:

> You have heard that it was said, 'You shall love your neighbor and hate your enemy.' But I say to you, Love your enemies and pray for those who persecute you so that you may be children of your Father in heaven ..." (Matt. 5:43-44)

It is easy to love those who love us. In some sense, Al Capone probably loved members of his immediate family. But Jesus' teachings consistently point beyond any limitations on love. When Jesus affirms that loving God and loving other people are the greatest commandments (Mark 12:28-34 par.), he also insists that his hearers expand their understanding of what it means to be "neighbor." The Parable of the Good Samaritan (Luke 10:29-37) delivers a tough message for his first-century fellow Jews; for this parable recognizes as "neighbor" and hence an object of love the group toward which they had the greatest hostility. Building upon the earlier love commands of Deuteronomy and Leviticus (Deut. 6:5; Lev. 19:18), Jesus *universalizes* the understanding of love.[25]

This teaching of expanded love directly addresses the needs of our current civilization of diverse peoples and traditions. The virtue of justice demands that we treat all people fairly. The virtue of love demands that we treat all people so that their greatest good will come about as a result of our interaction. From at least Thomas Aquinas forward, the Christian tradition has attempted to combine the four cardinal virtues (practical wisdom, justice, self-control, and courage) with the theological virtues (faith, hope, and love), the greatest of which is love. One of the most direct statements about divine character, "God is love" (1 John 4:8), implies an ethical goal for human character. If God is love, and we are to become the children of God, then we are to become the habitual practitioners of love.

While ethics always involves theory and instruction, the end of ethics is action. Saying that humankind must come to see itself as a planetary family does not magically solve the ethical issues of the global village. However, it does frame the issues; it provides a starting point for discussion. Decisions about what constitutes the good do not become automatic or easy. Real disagreements about the most substantive matters are unlikely to disappear. However, to the degree that love is adopted as an individual and collective goal, intelligent effort can be directed toward its achievement. In aiming to make love our second nature, "Would it not better equip us, like archers who have a target to aim at, to hit the proper mark?"[26] Similar to the way in which Aristotle would have us habituated into the Good, so too could we become habituated into practicing love. Love does not replace the other virtues, but it does situate them in a more comprehensive context.

Among those who share this kind of common goal, disagreements tend to be moderated by their placement within the larger familial context, a context that continues long after the disagreement. Family members do not always get along, let alone seek each other's highest good, but they recognize that they *ought* to do so. Members of a family, even those who have been separated by choice or by death, know that they are still family members. As a kind of *Weltanschauung*, the inescapable permanence of family relations provides a starting point for appreciating, making sense of, and, ultimately, through the practice of love, benefiting from the diversity in the planetary community. Believing ourselves the offspring of a common source and imagining a common destiny, our generation will have its own contribution to make in responding to the question of what human life means.

NOTES

1. Aristotle, *Nicomachean Ethics*, Translated with an Introduction by Martin Oswald (Indianapolis: Bobbs-Merrill, 1962), 1094b.
2. Aristotle, 1094a21.
3. Aristotle, 1094a24.
4. Aristotle, 1097b24.
5. What follows is my summation of the essence of Aristotle's argument in the *Nicomachean Ethics*.
6. Aristotle, without participating in anything like Judeo-Christian theism, seems at least to glimpse beyond the strictly human. In Book X of *Nicomachean Ethics*, he claims that man's highest activity is "contemplation"; for it imitates "most closely" "the activity of the divinity which surpasses all others in bliss" (1178b21).
7. For an excellent discussion of these four virtues, see Gilbert Meilaender, *The Theory and Practice of Virtue* (Notre Dame: University of Notre Dame Press, 1984).
8. This was the argument of the famous Sophist, Protagoras, whom Socrates attempts to refute. In the *Theaetetus*, when told that Protagoras had begun his discourse with, "Man is the measure of all things," Socrates humorously replies:

> I am surprised that he did not begin his *Truth* with the words, The measure of all things is the pig, or the baboon, or some sentient creature still more uncouth. There would have been something magnificent in so disdainful an opening, telling us that all the time, while we were admiring him for a wisdom more than mortal, he was in fact no wiser than a tadpole, to say nothing of any other human being.... If what every man believes as a result of perception is indeed to be true for him; if, just as no one is to be a better judge of what another experiences, so no one is entitled to consider whether what another thinks is true or false, and, ... every man is to have his own beliefs for himself alone and they are all right and true—then, my friend, where is the wisdom of Protagoras, to justify his setting up to teach others and to be handsomely paid for it, and where is our comparative ignorance or the need for us to go and sit at his feet, when each of us is himself the measure of his own wisdom? (*Theaetetus* 161c-e).

Socrates' target is *relativism*, a doctrine that still has many advocates, especially in college dormitories.

9. This was the position of the influential French sociologist, Emile Durkheim.
10. Friedrich Nietzsche, *The Will to Power* in *The Complete Works of Nietzsche*, O. Levy, ed. (New York: Macmillan, 1924), 200-201, as cited in *Vice and Virtue in Everyday Life: Introductory Readings in Ethics*, 4th ed., ed. Christina Sommers and Fred Sommers (Fort Worth: Harcourt Brace, 1997), 72.
11. John Milton, *Paradise Lost* I. 261-263, Norton Critical Edition, ed. Scott Elledge (New York: W.W. Norton and Co., 1975), 13.
12. Charles S. McCoy, *When gods Change: Hope for Theology* (Nashville: Abingdon, 1980), 99.

13. Michael Polanyi, *Personal Knowledge: Towards a Post-Critical Philosophy* (Chicago: University of Chicago Press, 1962), 195-202.
14. Polanyi, *Personal Knowledge*, 147.
15. Ibid., 403. For a further discussion of progress and how its achievement makes us more realistic, see my article, "Polanyi's Progress: Transcendence, Universality, and Teleology," in *Tradition and Discovery* XIX:2 (1993): 13-31, esp. 19.
16. Even the German term *"Weltanschauung"* does not escape this difficulty, since "Welt" is German for "world."
17. Thomas A. Langford, *Practical Divinity: Theology in the Wesleyan Tradition* (Nashville: Abingdon Press, 1983), 262.
18. Michael Novak, *The Spirit of Democratic Capitalism* (Lanham, Maryland: Madison Books, 1991), 39.
19. Huston Smith, *The World's Religions* (San Francisco: HarperSanFrancisco, 1991, revised and updated edition), 82.
20. Michael Polanyi, *Science, Faith, and Society* (Chicago and London: University of Chicago Press, 1946), 70.
21. Immanuel Kant, *Foundations of the Metaphysics of Morals*, trans. with an introduction by Lewis White Beck (Indianapolis: Bobbs-Merrill, 1959), 39, 47.
22. See, for example, "Idea for a Universal History from a Cosmopolitan Point of View," and "Perpetual Peace," in *On History*, The Library of Liberal Arts, edited and with an introduction by Lewis White Beck (New York: Macmillan Publishing Company, 1963).
23. Many Moslems are completely opposed to religiously motivated violence. Once again, the dividing line seems to be between exclusivistic and universalistic understandings of God.
24. See Jeffrey Wattles, *The Golden Rule* (New York, Oxford: Oxford University Press, 1996). Also see Wattles' article in this volume, "The Golden Rule Across the Curriculum."
25. See the article in this volume by W. Barnes Tatum, "Love As the Foundational Category for a Christian Ethic: From Command to Virtue."
26. Aristotle, *Nicomachean Ethics*, 1094a24.

QUESTIONS FOR DISCUSSION

1. Is "avoiding the bad" more than not being involved with harmful and injurious things?

2. Since ethics is never just a "me, myself, and I" business, what are the implications of a world that is shrinking as we become more connected through technology?

3. How are the cardinal virtues of practical wisdom, self-control, courage, and justice applicable in modern life?

4. What are the consequences of "choosing not to choose"?

5. Are all uses of power evil? Why or why not?

6. If our lives are gifts which our living should reflect through acts of gratitude, how do we do this? What does the gift of life have to do with responsibility? Obligation?

7. What does it mean to discover? To create? What are the differences and the implications of these differences?

8. Can truth change? How is acquiring new knowledge connected to truth?

PART ONE

CHRISTIAN ETHICS

LOVE AS THE FOUNDATIONAL CATEGORY FOR A CHRISTIAN ETHIC: FROM COMMAND TO VIRTUE

W. Barnes Tatum

ABSTRACT

The ethical stances of Catholic theologian Josef Pieper and Protestant theologian Reinhold Niebuhr, and the "Social Principles" of The United Methodist Church (1996), provide the framework for a consideration of love as the foundational category of a Christian ethic. The paper traces the trajectory of love, as a theological and ethical category, through nine stages. These stages extend from the social setting of love in ancient Israel as attested in the Hebrew Bible, through the use of love in the Pastoral Epistles which represent the emerging Gentile church in the wider Graeco-Roman world. Along the way, Israel's command ethic gives way to an emerging Hellenistic virtue ethic; and love itself makes the transition from command to virtue.

PREFACE: LOVE NOTES

"In contrast to symbiotic union, mature *love* is *union under the condition of preserving one's integrity*, one's individuality. *Love is an active power in man*; a power which breaks through the walls which separate man from his fellow man... . In love the paradox occurs that two beings become one and remain two." —Erich Fromm, *The Art of Loving* (1956)

And here's to you Mrs. Robinson,
Jesus loves you more than you will know (Wo wo wo)
God bless you please, Mrs. Robinson,
Heaven holds a place for those who pray (Hey hey hey hey hey hey)
— Paul Simon, "Mrs. Robinson" (1968)

"I love you, man!" —beer commercial (ca. 1997)

What's Love Got to Do With It (1993)
Color/119 minutes —Directed by Brian Gibson, and starring Angela Bassett and Laurence Fishburne as Tina Turner and Ike Turner

" 'GOD is love,' says St. John. When I first tried to write this book I thought that his maxim would provide me with a very plain high road through the whole subject. I thought I should be able to say that human loves deserved to be called loves at all just in so far as they resembled that Love which is God. The first distinction I made was therefore between what I called Gift-love and Need-love. The typical example of Gift-love would be that love which moves a man to work and plan and save for the future well-being of his family which he will die without sharing or seeing; of the second, that which sends a lonely or frightened child to its mother's arms." — C. S. Lewis, *The Four Loves* (1960)

"The most precious gift we can offer others is our presence. When our mindfulness embraces those we love, they will bloom like flowers. If you love someone but rarely make yourself available to him or her, this is not true love."
— Thich Nhat Hanh, *Living Buddha, Living Christ* (1995)

INTRODUCTION
CHRISTIAN THEOLOGY AND CHRISTIAN ETHICS

The Bible is neither a theological nor an ethical handbook. However, a Christian theology and a Christian ethic presuppose the Bible. Scripture serves as the basis for theological and ethical reflection.[1]

Throughout that portion of Christian Scripture known as the New–or Second–Testament, *love* appears as the recurring ethical category: in the four Gospels, in the genuine Letters of Paul, in the Letter of James, and even in the

Pastoral Epistles. Therefore, the title of this paper constitutes its thesis: *Love is the foundational category for a Christian ethic.*

To establish this thesis, I execute a "hermeneutical loop." I begin with brief comment on excerpts from the writings of two twentieth-century theological ethicists: Josef Pieper and Reinhold Niebuhr. I continue with an extensive, but not exhaustive, survey of Scriptural texts in their ancient literary and social contexts. Finally, I return to the twentieth century with further observations about the thought of Pieper and Niebuhr. I conclude by introducing, and commenting on, the "Social Principles" of The United Methodist Church (1996) and the "Universal Declaration of Human Rights," adopted by the General Assembly of the United Nations on December 10, 1948. The former offers additional support for the main thesis of the paper; and both provide bases for further ethical reflection.

PART ONE
JOSEF PIEPER AND REINHOLD NIEBUHR

The thought and writings of Josef Pieper (1904-1997) and Reinhold Niebuhr (1891-1979) provide examples of how love has functioned in recent Christian ethical reflection. Their writings also provide distinctively Catholic and Protestant expressions of a Christian ethic.

Josef Pieper, associated with the University of Münster, in Germany, for over half a century, has been one of the leading Thomistic thinkers of the present century, carrying forward the theological tradition of St. Thomas Aquinas (1225-1274).[2] In the brief, and readable, *What Catholics Believe: A Primer of the Catholic Faith*, Josef Pieper and his co-author Heinrich Raskop write:

> Virtue is not external good behavior and respectability. A good human being is a human in a higher manner than a bad one: he is in every respect more capable. Thus 'virtue' is the expression we use to describe the fact that man is exercising his essential abilities, that he is realizing his essential potentialities; that is, he is doing what is good, and not because he must but because he wants to and chooses to. ('Sin,' the deliberate turning away from God, means that man voluntarily becomes incapable of being and doing what is his true purpose to be and to do.) ...
>
> The most important of the Christian virtues are the three theological virtues and the four cardinal virtues. The three theological virtues are faith, hope, and love. The four cardinal virtues are prudence, justice, courage, and moderation.[3]

In traditional Catholic fashion, Pieper identifies love as a theological virtue along with faith and hope. Accordingly, these three virtues are realizable only in the life of a person who has experienced the sanctifying grace of the Triune God: Father, Son, Holy Spirit. The triad of theological virtues has its Scriptural basis in the New Testament writings of Paul. The four cardinal virtues represent the indebtedness of Catholic thought to Greek ethical tradition, especially to Aristotle (384-322 B.C.E.).

Reinhold Niebuhr, a professor for many years at Union Theological Seminary, in New York City, continues to be regarded by many as the leading American theologian of the twentieth century. In 1934, at Colgate-Rochester Seminary, Niebuhr gave the so-called Walter Rauschenbusch lectures. Walter Rauschenbusch, for whom the lectures were named, had been a leading proponent of the social gospel, that turn-of-the-century Protestant movement committed to applying the teachings of Jesus to the conditions of increasingly industrialized, urbanized society.[4]

Niebuhr used the occasion of these lectures to criticize what he perceived to be the ethical weaknesses not only of theological orthodoxy but also of theological liberalism. His lectures were published the next year, in 1935, as *An Interpretation of Christian Ethics*. In the preface to the 1956 edition of this volume, Niebuhr writes:

> The social gospel was that part of the liberal movement which had a sense of responsibility for social justice.. It thought that it could exercise that responsibility by insisting that love was the law of life in all and not merely in personal relations ....
>
> But there are many intricacies in the relation of love to justice. .... The primary issue is how it is possible to derive a social ethic from the absolute ethic of the gospels. The gospel ethic is absolute because it presents the final law of human freedom: the love of God and the neighbor. A social gospel must be concerned with the establishment of tolerable harmonies of life, tolerable forms of justice and tolerable stabilities in the flux of life. All this must be done, not by asking selfish people to love one another, neither by taking their self-love for granted. These harmonies must be established under "conditions of sin."[5]

Here Niebuhr claims that liberal theology was mistaken in its conviction that love could rule over social as well as personal relations. He also anticipates his own corrective. Given the complexity of social relations, he views justice as the expression of love in a world of competing political and economic interests. Nonetheless, like liberal theology and the social gospel he criticized, Niebuhr continues to identify love as the foundational category for a Christian ethic.

By contrast to the Catholic Josef Pieper, the Protestant Reinhold Niebuhr takes his ethical cue not from the theological virtues based on Paul and his Letters, but from the love commandment and the absolute ethic of the Gospels and Jesus. Nonetheless, both—as Christian theologians—take into account the ultimacy of God and the sinfulness of humankind in their ethical reflections.

PART TWO
SCRIPTURAL TEXTS AND CONTEXTS

Even a casual reading of the New Testament documents discloses that love appears therein as the pervasive ethical category. The Greek words underlying the word "love" in English translations of the New Testament are usually related to the Greek noun *agapē*, only occasionally to *philia*, and never to *erōs*.

Agapē, and its related forms, had been little used in classical Greek writings; but the Jewish translators of the Hebrew Bible into Greek (beginning in the third century B.C.E.) had used *agapē* to translate *'hb*, the Hebrew root for love. Therefore, not only the category of love but the vocabulary of love passed over into emerging Christianity from early Judaism by way of the Hebrew Bible and its translation into Greek, the Septuagint (LXX).

We begin our nine-stage survey of selected Scriptural texts with that section of the Christian canon known as the Old Testament. More specifically, we begin with the portion of the Old Testament known in the Hebrew Bible as the Torah.[6]

THE TORAH AND THE TEN COMMANDMENTS

The Torah (usually translated "law," more precisely meaning "instruction") consists of the five books of Moses: Genesis, Exodus, Leviticus, Numbers, Deuteronomy. The narrative begins with an account of how YHWH (the sacred, four-letter word for God) created the heavens and the earth and concludes with the death of Moses on a mountain overlooking the so-called promised land.

Critical scholarship considers the Torah to have reached its present form as late as the time of Ezra in the 400s B.C.E. through a complicated literary process that involved the weaving together of four major documentary sources or strands of tradition: J, E, D, P. Pre-exilic Israel and post-exilic Judaism represent the social matrix within which the Torah was fashioned; and the Torah itself narrates the formative history of YHWH's covenant people.

Within the Torah, several individual law codes have been identified, each with its own social and literary history. These codes include the following: the Ten Commandments (Exod. 20:1-17=Deut. 5:6-21); the Covenant Code (Exod. 20:22-22:23); the Holiness Code (Lev. 17–26); and the Deuteronomic Code (Deut. 5–28). Collectively, these codes constitute YHWH's requirements for YHWH's people. By their commitment to these commandments, YHWH's people distinguished themselves from the nations. The legal codes consist of individual commandments (*mitzvôth*). As early as the third century C.E., the commandments in the Torah were considered to number 613.[7] Given the multiplicity of commandments, there arose in Israel the attempt to identify general commandments or principles that epitomized the requirements of the entire Torah.

Some contemporary scholars have viewed that code known as the Ten Commandments (Exod. 20:1-17=Deut. 5:6-21), or Decalogue, as the oldest collection of commandments—dating, in its original form, from the time of Moses, in the 1200s B.C.E. However, other scholars have viewed the Decalogue as an attempt to epitomize the requirements of a more extensive legal tradition—post-Mosaic, but pre-exilic, before 587 B.C.E. The use of the Decalogue by Philo and Josephus, those great Hellenistic Jewish writers of the first century C.E., suggests that they considered the Decalogue as a summary statement of the entire Torah.[8] However, two commandments in the Torah, but outside the Decalogue, also came to serve an epitomizing function.

Two Commandments of Love
Leviticus 19:18 and Deuteronomy 6:5

Within the narrative setting of the Torah, Leviticus 19:18 represents a direct command given by YHWH through Moses to Israel during Israel's eleven-month sojourn at Mt. Sinai. Deuteronomy 6:5 also represents a command given by YHWH through Moses to Israel, but given during Israel's subsequent sojourn in the plains of Moab, east of the River Jordan.

The commandment in Deuteronomy 6:5 that calls for the love of YHWH has as its immediate literary setting the exhortation in Deuteronomy 6:4-9 that begins with the words: "Hear, O Israel." This stereotypical formula in Deuteronomy (see 5:1; 9:1; 20:3; 27:9) may have functioned in pre-exilic Israel as the traditional call for the tribes to gather for the worship of YHWH.

This commandment in Deuteronomy 6:5 requires a total love of YHWH that would express itself in specific religious practices. Within post-exilic Judaism, the words in Deuteronomy 6:4f became known as the *Sh^ema‘* literally "Hear," in Hebrew) and were recited regularly both by individuals and in corporate worship settings. Eventually, the words were taken literally, written down, and placed in phylacteries to be worn on the forehead and left arm and in mezuzahs to be fastened to doorposts.[9]

The commandment in Leviticus 19:18 appears in the midst of a hodgepodge collection of precepts that regulate daily life (19:1-37). Many of the precepts deal with agricultural matters. Others focus on interpersonal relations. The commandment in Leviticus 19:18 that calls for the love of "neighbor" (*rēa‘*) appears alongside other commandments (specifically, 19:15-18) that require right behavior toward "neighbor" (*rēa‘*), or "brother" (*’āh*), or your "people" (*’am*). Therefore, the love of neighbor in Leviticus 19:18 clearly mandates the love of a fellow Israelite.

However, the commandment in Leviticus 19:34 calls for the love of the "stranger" (*gēr*) who sojourns among the Israelites. Thus the circle of those to be loved includes non-Israelites. Furthermore, the criterion for love of the non-Israelite enjoined in Leviticus 19:34 is identical with the criterion for love of the neighbor set forth in Leviticus 19:18. Whether one loves a fellow Israelite or a non-Israelite, one loves that person as one loves oneself. Therefore, the criterion for loving others is self-love.

Furthermore, the collection of precepts about daily life (19:1-37) follows a detailed enumeration of forbidden sexual practices (18:1-30) and anticipates another listing of sexual offenses along with the required penalty—death (20:10-21). Just as the prohibition against killing (technically, against murder) excludes neither capital punishment nor holy war from the practices of ancient Israel (Exod. 20:13=Deut. 5:17), so the love of a neighbor does not exclude the execution of those who transgress the regulations of the covenant community.[10]

In the post-exilic period, the tendency to use general commandments, such as those in the Decalogue to epitomize the requirements of the entire Torah continued within Judaism. There is literary evidence. from as early as the second century B.C.E. that the two commandments to love YHWH and to love neighbor (Deut. 6:5 and Lev. 19:18) had been brought together and were already being used as an epitomizing summary of the Torah. The Testaments of the Twelve Patriarchs (T. Issachar 5:2 and T. Dan 5:3), among other writings, attest to this development.

The Golden Rule

Judaism did not confine itself to the commandments of the Torah to epitomize the Torah. Hillel, the first-century Pharisaic rabbi, reportedly was once approached by a Gentile. The Gentile promised to become a proselyte, or convert to Judaism, if Hillel could teach him the entire Torah while the Gentile stood on one foot. Hillel replied: "What is hateful to you, do not do to your neighbor; that is the whole Torah, while the rest is commentary thereon ... ."[11] Thus to epitomize the Torah, Hillel here uses a bit of wisdom virtually as old, and as universal, as humankind: the Golden Rule, albeit in its negative form.

Unlike the summary commandment in Deuteronomy 6:5, Hillel's version of the Golden Rule makes no mention of God. But like the summary commandment in Leviticus 19:18, Hillel's version refers to the neighbor. More importantly, like the commandment in Leviticus 19:18, the Golden Rule uses the individual self as the criterion for relating to others.

In his consideration of how the Golden Rule was expressed and used in Judaism, Jeffrey Wattles suggests that "golden rule thinking" is "predicated on the recognition that others are like oneself."[12] The same can be said of "love of neighbor thinking." Both require the ethical agent to place the self imaginatively in the other person's shoes.[13]

Not surprisingly, Jesus the first century Jew from Nazareth of Galilee reportedly used Deuteronomy 6:4f and Leviticus 19:18 as summary commandments, although he extends the scope of the latter commandment to encompass enemies. The Golden Rule also appears on Jesus' lips, but in its positive form: "In everything do to others as you would have them do to you" (Matt. 7:12); and "Do to others as you would have them do to you (Luke 6:31)."

The Great Commandment of Love
Mark 12:28-34 par.

The four canonical Gospels of Matthew, Mark, Luke, and John represent narratives of Jesus' life, especially his public activity as an adult. Critical scholarship, in spite of occasional dissenting alternatives, continues to consider Mark to be the earliest of these Gospels, written around 70 C.E.. Within a decade, the authors of Matthew and Luke had composed their Gospels using Mark as their principal written source. This use of Mark by Matthew and Luke accounts for the similarity among these so-called synoptic Gospels.

Among the stories about Jesus narrated by Mark is the one in which Jesus enters into dialogue with a scribe about the most important commandment in the Torah (12:28-34). In the Markan story, Jesus responds to the question about the most important commandment by citing, as had others before him, the two commandments to love YHWH (Deut. 6:4f) and to love neighbor (Lev. 19:18).

That these words of Jesus were actually spoken by him has been doubted by scholars who think the story reflects the effort by Mark and the earliest church to portray Jesus as a traditional Jewish teacher.[14] But there is a certainty: each of the synoptic authors has redacted, or edited, the story for that author's own purposes.[15]

Mark's version of the story serves an apologetic purpose for Gentiles who already believe the gospel about Jesus as the Christ. Jesus responds to the scribe by reciting the traditional *Sh^{e}ma'* with its emphasis on the oneness of God. Later in the dialogue, Jesus seemingly agrees with the scribe's claim that the love of God and the love of neighbor are superior to such religious acts as sacrifice. Both monotheism and philanthropy were ideas that Gentiles found attractive, first within Judaism and later within that Jewish movement that became Christianity.

Matthew's characteristically shortened version of the Markan story serves a polemical purpose. The interrogator of Jesus has become a lawyer from among the Pharisees. The lawyer, who approaches Jesus with malevolent intent, represents those non-believing Pharisees who stand in opposition to Matthew's own believing community that had itself come out of Pharisaic Judaism toward the end of the first century. Here there is no dialogue between the lawyer and Jesus. Jesus simply declares that the two love commandments, in Deuteronomy 6:5 and Leviticus 19:18, represent a summary of "all the Law and the Prophets"—a characteristically Jewish phrase that designates the two main divisions of Jewish Scripture (also Matt. 5:17 and 7:12).

Luke's radically altered version of the story serves a hortatory purpose for Gentiles who do not yet believe that Jesus is the Christ. The questioner, now identified simply as a lawyer, approaches Jesus not with the traditional Jewish question about the Torah but with the more universal question about eternal life. The two love commandments from Deuteronomy 6:5 and Leviticus 19:18 are melded together on the lips of the lawyer himself; and he sets Jesus up with another question: "And who is my neighbor?" Jesus answers by telling the parable of the Good Samaritan (Luke 10:29-37). The parable transforms the lawyer's question from "Who is my neighbor?" to "Toward whom must I show neighborliness?" In the parable, the Samaritan (the "other") demonstrates neighborliness whereas the priest and the Levite (the "religious officials") do not. Thus, in the Lukan narrative, the road from Jerusalem to Jericho has become the road to eternal life and neighborliness the vehicle that transports one to eternal life.

As noted, contemporary scholars have occasionally questioned whether Jesus himself used Deuteronomy 6:4f and Leviticus 19:18 to summarize the Torah; and even Luke in his narrative has removed these words from Jesus' lips. But scholars, virtually without dissent, acknowledge that the parable of the Good Samaritan confronts the hearer with the very voice of Jesus himself.[16] In the social world of first-century Palestine, Jesus with this parable undercuts both the ingrained hostility of Jews toward Samaritans as well as the traditional importance of temple worship and temple personnel.

Collectively, these three versions of the Great Commandment story contribute to "love of neighbor thinking" in several ways. Love of God and love of neighbor are inextricably related to one another. Together love of God and love of neighbor are preferable to religious, or cultic, acts. Indeed, love of God expresses itself in and through love of neighbor. Love of neighbor requires the ethical agent to imagine what neighborliness means in response to the immediate need of the other and to act accordingly. However, there is also a saying attributed to Jesus that takes the hearer even beyond "love of neighbor thinking."

LOVE OF ENEMIES
MATTHEW 5:44 AND LUKE 6:27, 35

Matthew and Luke, in addition to their use of Mark, also incorporate into their narratives extensive teaching material not found in Mark. Critical scholarship has come to identify this material common to Matthew and Luke by the symbol Q (from *Quelle*, German for "source"). In recent years, the view has reasserted itself that Q was a written document, Sayings Gospel Q.

In Matthew and Luke, there appears a remarkable Q saying where Jesus says: "love your enemies." This saying represents one about which there is the greatest degree of historical certainty.[17] But each Gospel writer has placed the saying in a narrative context peculiar to that Gospel. The author of Matthew places the saying within the context of the so-called Sermon on the Mount (5:1-7:29), in which Jesus sets forth a "righteousness" that exceeds that of the scribes and Pharisees (5:20). More specifically, the saying constitutes the last of the six antitheses in which Jesus quotes the Mosaic Torah and then offers his own contrasting teaching: "You have heard it was said .... But I say to you ... " (5:21-

48). The last antithesis reads: "You have heard it said, 'You shall love your neighbor and hate your enemy.' But I say to you, Love your enemies ... ." (5:43-44). The love of neighbor command, of course, represents the Leviticus 19:18 text prominent in Jewish discussions about the Torah. However, the hatred of enemy injunction occurs nowhere among the 613 commandments in the Torah. Nonetheless, Jesus is portrayed here as intentionally extending the scope of love beyond neighbor to include even enemies. Later in the Sermon on the Mount, Jesus also declares the Golden Rule (7:12), identified as a summary of "the Law and the Prophets" (compare 22:40).

The author of Luke has placed the love of enemies saying within the setting of the so-called Sermon on the Plain (6:17-49) in which Jesus addresses the crowds after his appointment of the twelve apostles. In fact, Jesus twice enjoins those gathered to love their enemies (6:27, 35). In each instance, Jesus immediately explains that loving enemies involves doing good to them. It is midway between these two love of enemy statements that Jesus declares the Golden Rule (6:31).

If "golden rule thinking" and "love of neighbor thinking" require a leap of the imagination, how much more does "love of enemy thinking"—along with a special act of the will! In Matthew and Luke, Jesus ultimately grounds his call for love of enemies in the recognition of God's universal beneficence. Thus, "love of enemy thinking" involves an imitation of God. In the Gospel of John, the imitation of God expresses itself as an imitation of Jesus Christ, the Son of God.

A NEW COMMANDMENT OF LOVE
JOHN 13:34 AND 15:13

The striking differences between the portrayal of Jesus in the synoptic Gospels and Jesus in the Gospel of John has resulted in the dominant scholarly view that the fourth Gospel is a theological affirmation in narrative form. In other words, the Gospel writer does not preserve what Jesus actually said, but has placed on Jesus' lips discourses that interpret the meaning of Jesus' life.[18]

Within the context of Jesus' farewell remarks at the last supper (13:1-17:26), Jesus says to his disciples: "I give you a new commandment, that you love one another. Just as I have loved you, you also should love one another" (13:34). By comparison with the Great Commandment reported in the Synoptics, this New Commandment in John is new in at least three ways.

First, the commandment is not derived from the Torah. Jesus quotes neither Deuteronomy 6:4f nor Leviticus 19:18.

Secondly, the criterion for loving others is not how people love themselves, but rather how Jesus has loved them. Earlier at the last supper in John, Jesus had given himself to the disciples by washing their feet. This act of self-giving both anticipates his own definitive act of self-giving on the cross and also serves as an example to be followed by his disciples. "New commandment thinking" presents an objective standard outside the self against which love can be measured. Not surprisingly, Jesus later gives what can be described as a corollary to the New Commandment: "No one has greater love than this, to lay down one's life for one's friends" (15:13).

Thirdly, the recipients of love are not neighbors, and certainly not enemies, but rather one another, those gathered in community around Jesus. Or, as the corollary states, believers lay down their lives for their friends (*philoi*). Therefore, in the Gospel of John, and in the Letters of John, love has an intramural dimension appropriate for a community of late first-century believers confronted and threatened by a hostile "world" (*kosmos*, an important category in these writings).

Nonetheless, this communal love is grounded in the very being, the universal intention, and the condescending act of God. God is love (1 John 4:16). God so loved the world that God gave the only Son, Jesus Christ (John 3:16). Jesus Christ loved his own who were in the world (John 13:1). Therefore, to imitate Jesus Christ is to imitate God, since Jesus Christ is the word of God made flesh (John 1:1,14).

Love as Commandment and as Virtue
Galatians 5:14 and 5:22

Thirteen letters in the New Testament present themselves as having been authored by Paul. Critical scholarship considers seven to be indisputably Pauline: Romans, 1 Corinthians, 2 Corinthians, Galatians, Philippians, 1 Thessalonians, and Philemon. Written by Paul to churches located in cities and towns along an arc stretching westward from Syria through Asia Minor and Greece to Italy, these letters probably date from the decade of the 50s C.E. They represent the earliest surviving documents from the nascent Christian movement.

Paul's letter to the Romans represents his longest, most systematic, theological presentation. As a sophisticated, Hellenized Jew, Paul knew the Torah—the Law. In the concluding ethical section of Romans (12:1-15:13), Paul cites Leviticus 19:18 as a summary of the Law: "You shall love your neighbor as yourself" (13:9).

The immediate context for this citation and its accompanying commentary (13:8-10) suggest that Paul understands "neighbor" (*plēsion*) to include those outside the circle of fellow believers. In fact, he has just articulated his position on the proper stance of believers, in Rome no less, toward "the governing authorities" (13:1-7)—that is, toward the Empire and toward Nero the Emperor (54-68 C.E.). By implication, Paul understands obedience to those in political power to be an expression of love.

Elsewhere in his correspondence, Paul also appeals to love as the basis for advice to his congregations on a variety of issues including meat offered to idols (1 Cor. 8:1-11:1) and tongues-speaking (1 Cor. 12:1-14:40), but not marriage (1 Cor. 7:1-40). His most powerful rhetorical use of love appears in his letter to Philemon involving the case of Onesimus, a runaway slave.

Paul cites Leviticus 19:18 as a summary of the Law not only in Romans but also in Galatians: "You shall love your neighbor as yourself" (5:14). But in the concluding ethical section of Galatians (5:1-6:10), we also see Paul's indebtedness to Hellenism. One of the characteristics of Greek ethical reflection was the listing of specific vices and virtues.[19] In Galatians, Paul juxtaposes lists of vices and virtues under the rubrics of "the works of the flesh" (5:19) and "the fruit of the Spirit" (5:22). For Paul, the fifteen vices represent those qualities that mark the human condition apart from Jesus Christ; and the nine virtues represent those qualities that mark a life "in Christ" or "in the Spirit" (to use characteristically Pauline phrasing). Here in Galatians, "love" heads the list of virtues followed by "joy, peace, patience, kindness, generosity, faithfulness, gentleness, and self-control."

Throughout Paul's writings, he associates love with faith and hope (e.g., 1 Thess. 1:3; 5:8). Collectively, this triad serves as a brief, but comprehensive, way for Paul to summarize what it means to be "in Christ." He places the positive categories of faith, love, and hope over against the negative categories of sin, law, and death.

In 1 Corinthians 13, Paul (ironically remembered in Protestantism as the apostle of faith) concludes his tribute to love with this declaration: "And now faith, hope, and love abide, these three; and the greatest of these is love." Paul's elevation of love above the other categories stems from his association of love not only with human responsibility but with the nature of God. Although not as focused in this regard as the author of John, Paul celebrates the love of God in the central section of Romans with its hymnic conclusion (5:1-8:39).

LOVE AS THE ROYAL LAW
JAMES 2:8

The Letter of James was written possibly toward the end of the first century. This document, more of a treatise than a letter, may have been written in conscious opposition to Paul's teaching on justification by faith, although the author of James may have had a distorted view of Paul's teaching. Nonetheless, in order to emphasize "works," the author also cites the love commandment in Leviticus 19:18 as binding on believers of Jesus Christ. He even refers to the commandment to love one's neighbor as "the royal law" (2:8). By contrast, the Pastoral Epistles no longer anchor love in Scripture; and love no longer functions as the central and overriding ethical category. Love has become one virtue among many.

LOVE AS A VIRTUE
THE PASTORAL EPISTLES

The so-called Pastoral Epistles (1 Timothy, 2 Timothy, and Titus) constitute a subgroup of letters claiming to have been written by Paul to his most trusted co-workers. In all probability, these letters were written by someone from a later generation who admired Paul. The author wrote, using Paul's name, to define what constituted right teaching, right belief, and right behavior for a later day and time.

No writings in the New Testament give more evidence of Christian communities making themselves at home in the Graeco-Roman world than do the Pastorals. These Letters draw upon conventional morality to identify those virtues to be exhibited and those vices to be avoided both by church leaders and by the rank-and-file participants. Lists of virtues and vices abound, especially vices (e.g., 1 Tim. 1:9-10; 6:4-5; 2 Tim. 3:2-5; Titus 3:3).

Although the traditional Pauline categories of faith and love are often linked in the Pastorals, they appear alongside other virtues and are not accorded any prominence. Furthermore, faith and love are associated with two of the four cardinal virtues of Greek ethical tradition: "justice" (*dikaiosunē*) and "moderation" (*sōphrosunē*).

The Paul of the Pastorals extols his own virtues: "... my teaching, my conduct, my aim in life, my faith, my patience, my love, my steadfastness ... ." (2 Tim. 3:10-11). Paul also exhorts Timothy to seek "righteousness, godliness, faith, love, endurance, gentleness" (1 Tim. 6:11). And Paul directs Titus to teach others that they must be "temperate, serious, sensible, and sound in faith, in love, and in endurance." (Titus 2:2).

Love entered the earliest church in Palestine as a verb, by way of Deuteronomy 6:4f and Leviticus 19:18 and through the teaching of Jesus. But in a religious community struggling to establish itself in the wider world of the Roman Empire, love became a noun—through the assistance of Greek moral philosophy. Along the way, the church made the transition from Judaism to Hellenism, from Jew to Gentile, from commandment to virtue. In retrospect, the Pastoral Epistles stand on the Hellenistic/Gentile/virtue side of the divide and represent what would become a catholic (from Greek for "universal") church.

PART THREE
JOSEF PIEPER AND REINHOLD NIEBUHR

As the pervasive ethical category throughout the New Testament, *love became the foundational ethical category for a Christian ethic*. The double legacy of love as virtue and as command has expressed itself along Catholic and Protestant trajectories of ethical reflection.

The Catholic ethic of Josef Pieper, in the Thomistic tradition, emphasizes love as a virtue—a theological virtue that finds its Scriptural warrant in the teaching of Paul. The ethic of Reinhold Niebuhr, with an indebtedness to Protestant liberalism, emphasizes love as a commandment—an absolute commandment that finds its Scriptural warrant in the uncompromising message of Jesus.

CONCLUSION
"SOCIAL PRINCIPLES" AND "HUMAN RIGHTS"

The theological liberalism to which Niebuhr was responding in his 1934 Rauschenbusch lectures had already prompted Protestant denominations to articulate position statements on the relationship between the gospel and social issues. In 1908, the Methodist Episcopal Church became the first denomination to adopt such a statement. That brief, less than one page, statement concerned itself exclusively with economic issues. Every four years since then, what has become The United Methodist Church has revised its statement in the light of new theological insights and changing social issues.

The current "Social Principles" of The United Methodist Church was adopted by the General Conference in 1996. Now thirty-four pages in length, the statement addresses virtually all areas of ethical concern: the natural world, the family, the social community, the economic community, and the world community. The United Methodist statement is not of importance because of its normative status as far as particular ethical positions are concerned—even for United Methodists. But the statement is important because it illustrates the kind of positions taken on ethical issues by churches in a modern, or postmodern, world.

The "Social Principles" of The United Methodist Church has a counterpart in the "Universal Declaration of Human Rights" (1948) adopted by the General Assembly of the United Nations. The opening words of the preamble of this latter statement declare: "Whereas recognition of the inherent and of the equal and inalienable rights of all members of the human family is the foundation of freedom, justice, and peace in the world ... ." The United Nations statement itself consists of thirty articles that spell out human rights pertaining to all areas of life: political, economic, family, etc. Like the Methodist statement, therefore, this document claims that all humans *as humans* have certain rights. Like the Methodist statement, this document dares to spell out these rights in some detail. However, I prefer the United Methodist statement over the United Nations declaration. The preamble of the "Social Principles" recognizes love to be the foundation for universal human community. The preamble also makes it clear that the presupposition and basis for the community of love into which all persons are called is the love of God (italics are mine):

> We, the people called United Methodists, affirm our faith in God our Creator and Father, in Jesus Christ our Savior, and in the Holy Spirit, our Guide and Guard.
>
> We acknowledge our complete dependence upon God in birth, in life, in death, and in life eternal. Secure in *God's love*, we affirm the goodness of life and confess our many sins against God's will for us as we find it in Jesus Christ. We have not always been faithful stewards of all that has been committed to us by God the creator. We have been reluctant followers of Jesus Christ in his mission to bring *all persons into a community of love*. Though called by the Holy Spirit to become new creatures in Christ, we have resisted the further call to become the people of God in our dealings with each other and the earth on which we live. Grateful for *God's forgiving love*, in which we live and by which we are judged, and affirming our belief in the inestimable worth of each individual, we renew our commitment to become faithful witnesses to the gospel, not alone to the ends of the earth, but also to the depths of our common life and work.
>
> —Preamble, "Social Principles,"
> The United Methodist Church (1996)

NOTES

1. The use of Scripture by eight theological ethicists has recently been analyzed by Jeffrey Siker, *Scripture and Ethics: Twentieth-Century Portraits* (New York and Oxford: Oxford University Press, 1997).
2. Especially: St. Thomas Aquinas, *Treatise on the Virtues*, trans. John A. Oesterle (Notre Dame, IN: University of Notre Dame Press, 1984).
3. Josef Pieper and Heinrich Raskop, *What Catholics Believe: A Primer of the Catholic Faith*, trans. Jan van Heurck (Chicago: Franciscan Herald Press, 1983), 59-60.
4. Especially: Walter Rauschenbusch, *A Theology for the Social Gospel* (1917; Nashville and New York: Abingdon Press, 1945).
5. Reinhold Neibuhr, *An Interpretation of Christian Ethics* (New York: Meridian Books, 1956), viii-xi.
6. The Scriptural quotations in this paper are based on the New Revised Standard Version (1989). This paper presupposes the commonly held literary theories with regard to the Hebrew Bible, or Old Testament, and the New Testament. These include the four-source. hypothesis for the Torah (J, E, D, P) and the two-source hypothesis for the Gospels (Mark and Q). For discussions of these and other critical viewpoints presented in this paper, consult any of the standard introductory textbooks, such as, Barry L. Bandstra, *Reading the Old Testament: An Introduction to the Hebrew Bible* (Belmont, CA: Wadsworth, 1995); Bernard W. Anderson, *Understanding the Old Testament*, abridged, 4th ed. (Upper Saddle River, NJ: Prentice-Hall, 1998); David L. Barr, *New Testament Story: An Introduction*, 2nd ed. (Belmont, CA: Wadsworth, 1994); Stephen L. Harris, *The New Testament: A Student's Introduction*, 2nd ed. (MountainView, CA: Mayfield, 1995).
7. All 613 commandments are easily accessible, listed according to the enumeration of the great medieval Jewish philosopher Moses Maimonides (1135-1204): I. Broydé, "Commandments, The 613," *The Jewish Encyclopedia* (New York and London: Funk and Wagnalls, 1903), IV, 181-186.
8. Cited in W. Barnes Tatum, "The LXX Version of the Second Commandment (Ex 20:3-6=Deut 5:7-10): A Polemic Against Idols, not Images," *Journal for the Study of Judaism* XVII, no.2 (1986):178-195.
9. Gerhard Von Rad, *Deuteronomy* (Philadelphia: Westminster Press, 1966), 62-65.
10. Martin Noth, *Leviticus* (Philadelphia: Westminster Press, 1965), 136-144.
11. Cited in Jeffrey Wattles, *The Golden Rule* (New York and Oxford: Oxford University Press, 1996), 48.
12. Ibid., 44.
13. Ibid., 105-121.
14. For example, Robert W. Funk, Roy Hoover, and the Jesus Seminar, *The Five Gospels* (New York: Macmillan, 1993), 104-105. But compare Reginald H. Fuller, "The Double Commandment of Love: A Test Case for the Criteria of Authenticity," in *Essays on the Love Commandment* (Philadelphia: Fortress Press, 1978), 9-39.
15. Victor Paul Furnish, *The Love Command in the New Testament* (Nashville and New York: Abingdon, 1972), 70-90; also W. Barnes Tatum, *In Quest of Jesus: A Guidebook* (Louisville, KY: Westminster/John Knox Press, 1982), passim.
16. Funk, *Five Gospels*, 323-324.

17. Ibid., 145-147, 291. Exactly what Jesus meant by the love of enemies saying is less than certain. Richard A. Horsley has argued that the "enemies" referred to by Jesus, within the social setting of his grassroots activity, were neither foreign enemies such as the Romans nor political enemies such as the priestly establishment. Jesus was addressing peasants in small villages caught in desperate social and economic circumstances. They had become enemies to each other. Although Horsley concludes by considering the implications of his study for contemporary approaches to ethics, he denies that Jesus' saying originally addressed the larger issues of pacifism or non-violence. See his "Ethics and Exegesis: 'Love Your Enemies' and the Doctrine of Non-Violence," *Journal of the American Academy of Religion* LIV, no.1 (1986): 3-31.

18. Tatum, *In Quest of Jesus*, 52-59.

19. On lists of virtues and vices, see Wayne A. Meeks, *The Origins of Christian Morality: The First Two Centuries* (New Haven and London: Yale University Press, 1993); and his *Moral World of the First Christians* (Philadelphia: Westminster Press, 1986).

QUESTIONS FOR DISCUSSION

1. What is the Golden Rule? What is the Great Commandment? What is the New Commandment? Which of these three commandments grows out of universal human experience? Which has its origin within ancient Israel and early Judaism? Which has its origin within emerging Christianity?

2. Is self-love a prerequisite for the Golden Rule? Can a person love his/her neighbor if that person lacks self-love?

3. What does it mean to say that "golden rule thinking" requires a specific act of the will?

4. What does it mean to say that "love of enemy thinking" requires a special act of the will? What can we learn by examining our loving actions aimed toward our enemies?

5. How can "love of neighbor thinking" and "love of enemy thinking" inform our private and public lives? What about capital punishment? What about war?

6. How do the ethical statements by Josef Pieper and Reinhold Neibuhr resemble and differ from each other?

7. How does the Methodist statement of "Social Principles" differ from the United Nations "Universal Declaration of Human Rights"?

ETHICS IN METHODISM

Thomas A. Langford

ABSTRACT

Methodism as a Christian tradition has been characterized by its effort to hold theology and ethics together. The two are inseparable and interactive: theology is intended to underwrite practices, and life-engagement guides theological interpretation. Persistent pressures attempt to divide the two; theology is tempted to become abstract or self-contained and ethical action is tempted to become independent of theological bases. Nevertheless, this tradition has its distinctive character in its continual attempt to understand the roots of action in God's incarnate life and to express its theological conviction in authentic Christian living. For this reason Methodism has endeavored to follow the lead of its founder John Wesley in producing a practical theology.

What is the role of ethics in Methodist thought and life? This question is not one that asks for proof that Methodism is unique or that contrasts Methodism with other Christian traditions in order to prove its superiority. Rather it is to describe the role of ethics in the Methodist tradition.[1]

For Methodism, the understanding of moral responsibility is rooted in its founder John Wesley, an eighteenth-century church leader who held theory and practice in tight tension. Theory, to be significant, is worked out in practice, and practice contributes to and enriches theory. Both are necessary. Each is incomplete without the other. For Wesley the combination was crucial because he was not so interested in interpreting the world as he was in transforming it. While insightful interpretation might be necessary for effective transformation, both his basis for interpretation and the goals sought in transformation were rooted in a Christian understanding of life in God.

JOHN WESLEY'S PRACTICAL THEOLOGY

Wesley understood himself to be a practical theologian. That is, true Christian understanding is reached when life is an expression of this conviction. The time-honored distinction between faith and works is overridden by the close interaction of the two. Faith is expressed in works; works reveal one's faith. Theory and practice are inseparable; theology and ethics live together.

To say, for Wesley, "I believe," is to express one's way of being, the fundamental character of one's way of living. Faith is not simply or exclusively a mental or rational belief, it is also an expression of affective (emotional) love, a volitional (willful) affirmation and a response which leads directly to action. Faith that does not shape life is false faith; action that does not conform to its primary affirmation is false action. "False" in both cases means inauthentic, artificial, unfulfilled, unrooted.

There have been debates over whether Wesley's social practices are derived from his theology (Schneeberger) or whether his theology is derived from his social ethic (Marquardt). That an answer is difficult illustrates the tight binding by which the two are held together.

What were Wesley's theological foundations? What were his practical ethical actions? Wesley rooted his theology in a doctrine of grace: grace free to all and free for all. Grace, for Wesley, is a person: grace is Jesus Christ; Jesus Christ is grace. This person conveyed the reach of God to establish positive relationship with human beings and to establish positive relationship among human beings. God's action becomes the cause and character of those who become disciples of Jesus Christ.

God's grace is the giving of God's self. Grace is offered freely, without preconditions. It is expressed as judgment on false relationships either with God or other human beings (i.e., judgment itself is understood as an act of grace which attempts to reorder and reform life). It seeks out those in special need. Its goal is reconciliation. And it is steadfast and unfailing.

In terms of types of ethical theory, how should Wesley's position be characterized? He, of course, did not use these categories, but is he more like one who obeys explicit demands (deontology)? Is he end-directed to commanding goals (teleology)? Is he a utilitarian seeking the greatest good for the greatest number? Or is he a eudaemonist (affirmation of happiness in life) seeking joy and fulfillment for human beings?

Wesley did not think in these terms. But, if pushed, he would probably say that his position was a mixture of all of these. There are commands of

God; love should respond to love. There are ends to be served, the transforming of human life in community with God. This transformation should seek to extend this good to the greatest number of people. And, by following this way, human happiness is truly found.

Wesley's emphases tie all of these themes together. No one theme possesses exclusive priority over the others. The true base of his thought is human life rooted in the life of God in Jesus Christ. Ethics is the extension of this primary and shaping relationship in all relationships

Wesley stressed the notion of "The Imitation of Christ." Christians are to attempt, in their necessarily limited ways, to embody the qualities of Christ's life in their love of God and love of neighbor. He recommended that his followers read the biographies of saintly Christians. To promote this reading, Wesley produced *A Christian Library*, a fifty-volume set of books. Forty-eight of the volumes were composed of stories of people who provided concrete examples for saintly living. Wesley built his theological foundation upon the New Testament witness: You are to love one another as I have loved you (John 13:34).

In his time, Wesley found ethical expression in meeting particular issues. He opposed slave trading and slavery; he was constantly concerned about those who were in poverty (in his ninety-first year he went out in the snow to collect money for the poor); he was opposed to smuggling (which was common on the coast); and he spoke against personal habits which represented disregard of others. Morality was extremely concrete. Wesley wanted to meet actual conditions in a Christian spirit so as to effect change.

Wesley felt especially called to minister to ordinary workers and tradespeople. He preached out of doors in order to meet these people where they were. When he traveled, he did not stay in manor houses or with gentry. He did not establish chapels in the five richest boroughs of London. He continually arranged for help to be given to widows and children. He stressed literacy and personal education.

It is not without significance that the Salvation Army, founded in the mid-nineteenth century, was an offshoot of Methodism. It is not coincidental that Methodism was working in inner city life, on workers' status, or was concerned about the general condition of the people.

Historians who evaluate the Wesleyan movement range from those who say that it so changed conditions in England that it prevented a "French Revolution" (Halevy) to those who maintain that it reinforced the status quo (E.P.Thompson). Both arguments acknowledge that the Wesleyan movement had a seminal influence on British life.

In many ways Wesley's ethical concerns were more noted than his theology. But the truer picture insists on the inseparability of the two. Each implies the other, each fulfills the other.

WESLEY'S SUCCESSORS

Methodism expanded rapidly in the nineteenth century. It became a world movement, following the roads and the reach of the British Empire. We shall follow its lead to the North American continent.

In 1784 John Wesley sent Francis Asbury and Thomas Coke to the United States to establish the Methodist Church in North America. Through their efforts, Asbury and Coke created a movement which continued Wesley's theological and ethical concerns. But in this ensuing tradition practical matters of application often became more prominent than did attention to theological underpinnings. On the North American scene people often spoke of Methodists as being "pragmatic"; that is, the movement was sensitive to its social setting and gave primary attention to achieve practical ways of being morally responsible in and for their society.

METHODISM IN AMERICA

Nineteenth-century Methodism in North America was initially a counter-cultural movement. Methodists opposed the flaunting of affluence. They protested against the faddishness of style; they were strict sabbatarians. They did not wear jewelry or makeup; preachers dressed in black broadcloth suits; and women wore dresses high at the neck, low at the hem. They advised their members not to go to the theater, play cards, play games on Sunday, drink alcohol or smoke. These counter-cultural moves were calculated to help followers keep basic priorities straight. Wesley's theme was extended into the next generation: do all the good you can, in every way you can, for as long as you can.

As the nineteenth century progressed, Methodism became a more potent social force. From no appearance on the 1770 national census, it became the largest religious body in the nation by 1825. Winthrop Hudson, a Baptist American historian, has claimed that the period from 1825 until the First World War was "The Methodist Age" in the United States. In the middle of this period, Methodism split over slavery and contributed more soldiers to both sides of the conflict than any other religious group. In this era Methodism was strongly identified with workers, women and children.

In 1908 a famous "Social Creed" (Appendix I) was adopted and was required reading in every congregation. It was a political manifesto which stressed such themes as the right of workers to form unions, the limitation of the hours of the work week, and the need for child labor laws.

By this time, Methodism clearly expressed its concern for the lower and lower middle-class segments of the population. This church was the church of ordinary people. Its members continued to be suspicious of wealth, of social hierarchy and of secular values. (It is instructive that Methodism built its educational institutions for ordinary lay people, not especially for clergy or for the social elite.) This was an egalitarian movement.

Methodist preachers and theologians were especially attentive to the particular social and intellectual climate in which they lived. Intellectually this meant that Methodist theologians attempted to use dominant philosophical convictions to present their faith. From the late nineteenth century, when Borden Parker Bowne used philosophical idealism (and created a school known as Boston Personalism) through liberal social gospel interests (shared with Walter Rauschenbusch and other North American Protestants) in the early decades of this century, Methodism was engaged with its cultural context. So Carl Michalson worked with existentialist philosophy and Schubert Ogden and John B. Cobb, Jr., with process thought. All of these theologians were concerned to present the gospel in such a way that their contemporaries could understand, assimilate and be transformed by it.

A sharp ethical focus was realized in the second half of the present century as Methodist theologians concentrated on special conditions of oppression that limit and defraud human life. For instance, James Cone develops themes of Black theology, Rebecca Chopp speaks from a feminist perspective and Theodore Jennings has related Methodism to liberation concerns.

In North America, Methodism was better known for its social activism than for its underlying theology. By mid-twentieth century, the church was exceedingly broad, probably more inclusive of diverse social, economic, educational and racial groupings than any other Protestant denomination. Some groups moved toward radical social restructuring, such as The Methodist Federation for Social Action (which brought a false charge in the *Reader's Digest* under the title, "Methodism's Pink Fringe.") Other groups, such as Good News and the "Confessing Movement" were formed to counter progressive social engagement and reaffirm traditional moralities.

Within the church these struggles also took the form of different theological interests, such as the primacy of scripture or experience, or the primacy of theory or practice. The issues have moved back and forth from priority to exclusion. Faith and works have often collided.

Discussion of the function of "faith" has tended to raise the question of why we should be moral. The function of "works" concentrates on how we can be moral. The reason for acting ethically is rooted in one's primary faith commitment: as disciples of Jesus Christ, we are to attempt to embody the mind and spirit of Jesus Christ; we act as we do because of how God has acted. This motivation frames our intentions and actions. These are theological considerations.

To concentrate on "works" is to ask how love may be expressed most adequately, most helpfully, and most lastingly. These are practical questions, questions of social policy, of sensitive benevolence, and of personal maturity. These questions can be served by social sciences and by experimental testing.

This short history emphasizes the fact that Methodism has been socially sensitive, an ongoing effort to speak directly and morally about personal and social conditions. Among Methodists, but not exclusive to Methodists, there developed in mid-century a special area of studies called "social ethics." This interest has been well represented by such people as Walter Muelder, Philip Wogaman and Clint Gardner. Further subdivisions have developed as ethics became more specialized as medical ethics and business ethics, for instance. A combination of ethics and theology has continued with these writers, but primary weight is given to ethical outputs.

By continually updating its "Social Creed" (Appendix II) and through its organized church programs, The United Methodist Church (founded by Methodist traditions coming together in 1968) has continued to express ethical concerns. The relation between theory and practice, however, has been difficult to achieve or maintain. Over the last two centuries more attention has been paid to applying the faith than to investigating the roots of the faith. In recent decades there has been a resurgence of holding theology and ethics together, of insisting that they must be seen as inseparably connected, as each requiring and fulfilling the other. Several people have played significant roles in this effort, such as Paul Ramsey, who fought both relativism and utilitarianism; Thomas Ogletree; and, contemporarily, Stanley Hauerwas. These persons understand themselves to be theological ethicists who place primary emphasis upon the theological bases for ethical theory and practice.

Contemporarily, United Methodism lives with sharp awareness of the globalization of life, the clash of cultures, the struggles for reconciliation among peoples, races, and nations, and the economically and politically marginalized people. Methodism is now world-wide. "What about Methodism," E. Gordon Rupp asked in a conversation, "which covers the world a quarter of an inch thick?"

As Methodism confronts the world as a religious minority, it is challenged to make its own distinctive but not unique, contribution as a holistic expression of faith-life. It must also learn to find common cause with other traditions as the well being of society is sought. Distinctive yet cooperative life is an enduring theme.

CONCLUSION

Theories are many, practices are diverse, the challenge is profound. Intellectual and ethical responsibility is placed upon all Christians and Methodists to participate in the ongoing effort to establish foundations for, and to explore creative expressions of, Christian discipleship.

Theology and practice, or more aptly, theological practice or practical theology, characterized the origin of this Methodist movement. The relationship is tender and has often been overbalanced, usually in the direction of application. But the times are constantly changing and each new generation has responsibility for interpreting the mind and spirit of Jesus Christ in order to achieve its own faithful witness.

NOTES

1. More complete reference to the people and ideas discussed in this essay may be found in Thomas A. Langford, *Practical Divinity: Theology in the Wesleyan Tradition*, 2nd ed. (Nashville: Abingdon Press, 1998).

SUGGESTED READINGS

Chopp, Rebecca S. *The Power to Speak.* New York: Crossroad, 1992.

Cobb, John B. Jr., *Grace and Responsibility: A Wesleyan Theology for Today.* Nashville: Abingdon, 1995.

Hauerwas, Stanley. *The Peaceable Kingdom.* Notre Dame, IN: Notre Dame, 1983.

Heitzenrater, Richard P. *Wesley and The People Called Methodists.* Nashville: Abingdon, 1995.

Langford, Thomas A. *Practical Divinity: Theology in the Wesleyan Tradition,* 2nd ed. Nashville: Abingdon, 1998.

Outler, Albert C., ed. *John Wesley.* New York: Oxford, 1980.

APPENDIX I

SOCIAL CREED, 1908

The Methodist Episcopal Church stands-

For equal rights and complete justice for all men in all situations of life, For the principle of conciliation and arbitration in industrial dissensions.
For the protection of the worker from dangerous machinery, occupational diseases, injuries and mortality.
For the abolition of child labor.
For such regulation of the conditions of labor for women as shall safeguard the physical and moral health of the community.
For the suppression of the "sweating system."
For the gradual and reasonable reduction of the hours of labor to the lowest practical point, with work for all; and for that degree of leisure for all which is the condition of the highest human life.
For a release from employment one day in seven. For a living wage in every industry.
For the highest wage that each industry can afford and for the most equitable division of the products of industry that can ultimately be devised.
For the recognition of the Golden Rule and the mind of Christ as the supreme law of society and the sure remedy for all social ills.

Taken from *the Journal of the Methodist Episcopal Church* (1908).

APPENDIX II

OUR SOCIAL CREED

We believe in God, Creator of the world; and in Jesus Christ, the Redeemer of creation. We believe in the Holy Spirit, through whom we acknowledge God's gifts, and we repent of our sin in misusing these gifts to idolatrous ends.

We affirm the natural world as God's handiwork and dedicate ourselves to its preservation, enhancement, and faithful use by humankind.

We joyfully receive for ourselves and others the blessings of community, sexuality, marriage, and the family.

We commit ourselves to the rights of men, women, children, youth, young adults, the aging, and people with disabilities; to improvement of the quality of life; and to the rights and dignity of racial, ethnic, and religious minorities.

We believe in the right and duty of persons to work for the glory of God and the good of themselves and others and in the protection of their welfare in so doing; in the rights to property as a trust from God, collective bargaining, and responsible consumption; and in the elimination of economic and social distress.

We dedicate ourselves to peace throughout the world, to the rule of justice and law among nations, and to individual freedom for all people of the world.

We believe in the present and final triumph of God's Word in human affairs and gladly accept our commission to manifest the life of the gospel in the world. Amen.

Taken from *The Book of Discipline of the United Methodist Church* (Nashville: United Methodist Publishing House, 1996).

QUESTIONS FOR DISCUSSION

1. Socrates believes that to know the good is to be the good is to do the good. How is this similar to or different from John Wesley's "Practical Theology"?

2. John Wesley faced slavery, poverty, and smuggling. What current issues do we face today? How can we meet these conditions with a Christian spirit and with a reforming outcome?

3. What does is mean to be morally responsible?

4. In today's society, how might we apply John Wesley's theme: "Do all the good you can, in every way you can, for as long as you can"?

5. Do you think the 1908 Social Creed would be adopted in the Modern Church?

THE GOLDEN RULE ACROSS THE CURRICULUM

Jeffrey Wattles

ABSTRACT

Education promotes success and growth. Growth involves service, and service involves the practice of the golden rule. The principle, Do to others as you want others to do to you, deserves study and application throughout our educational system, on moral and religious grounds.

Every academic discipline can contribute to the goal of character growth, where character is understood as the love of service, and service is understood as the practice of the golden rule: Do to others as you want others to do to you. It makes a difference when a professor teaches with the primary goal of bringing good to the student; and it makes a difference when a student pursues education with the primary goal of preparing for service.

One of the most widely recognized principles in the character education movement is that right actions are essential to character growth. As the proverb goes, "Sow an action, reap a habit. Sow a habit, reap a character. Sow a character, reap a destiny." In other words, it is not enough to read about character and discuss service; it is necessary to become morally active.

Many students are becoming morally active, due in part to the fact that more and more schools, including high schools, are requiring a certain number of service hours as a graduation requirement. In the growing service-learning movement, service becomes an integral part of class work. Community service organizations are the most common places in which students perform service for that component of their courses. Nevertheless, the community service model should not obscure the fact that service is properly an affair that pervades the whole of life; so in my philosophy classes I give my students a wide range of choice of service projects. I often suggest that students select an approach to an assigned paper that will enable them not merely to fulfill an assignment but also to bring good to someone else. Sometimes I assign a term project in which the student is to choose an issue and choose a person, group, or institution for interaction throughout the term. The research and writing relates to that interaction; as the term progresses, specific paper assignments enable the student to reflect on personal experience. I often ask for a one-page experience report, followed by a couple of pages in which the student is asked to comment on that experience from the perspective of the author of the text we are studying, followed by the student's comments on that author's perspective. The final paper to be handed in is a copy of what the student has sent to his or her person, group, or institution in an effort to make a contribution.

The golden rule can be practiced in any academic field, and many disciplines have specific contributions to offer on the meanings and values of the golden rule. For example, the rule is commonly associated with the recommendation to put oneself "in the other person's shoes," in other words, to imagine the other's situation from that person's perspective. Consider the importance of empathy in human interaction and the challenges of gaining a good understanding of other people, especially those that differ from us in important ways. Biology, social sciences, and the humanities all have contributions to make in the adventure of coming to understand ourselves and others.

THE ECLIPSE OF THE GOLDEN RULE
IN CONTEMPORARY ACADEMIC ETHICS

The golden rule, which did not get its modern name until the seventeenth century, had a complex origin in the cultures of the ancient world. For some fourth century BCE Greek sophists formulas akin to the rule expressed a handy technique for getting along smoothly with people; three centuries later the rule entered Jewish literature and began to function as a summary of Jewish religious ethics. The rule was used to symbolize the hierarchical demands of Chinese society and the moral teachings of Jesus. In each tradition, despite their diversity, the practice of the golden rule and reflection on it seems to have led to growth in insight and interpretation. One reason for the widespread appeal of the rule is that any person, no matter what his or her level of moral development, can immediately make sense of it and begin to apply it; and practice with the rule brings higher meanings and values to light.[1]

Given the widespread popularity of the golden rule, why is there a comparative lack of appeal to it in academic ethics? In some cases—most notably that of Immanuel Kant in the *Grounding of the Metaphysics of Morals*[2]—reflection on the golden rule has led thinkers to raise problems. Kant said that the golden rule is incomplete in failing to provide a basis for duties to oneself. He objected that no universal or rigorous sense of duty could be derived from a principle that appeals to the way the agent wants to be treated. True, the golden rule is worded in a way suited to the needs of most people most of the time, but not in a way suited for use in the most rigorous moral reasoning. As a modern philosopher or theologian raises an objection to the rule, he or she faces a choice among three options: (1) to abandon the rule, as did Paul Tillich, for example; (2) to reformulate the rule (as I believe Kant did in the categorical imperative) in order to construct a formulation that is invulnerable to the objection; (3) to make use of the objection to develop a more mature, inclusive, and flexible interpretation of the rule as commonly worded.

Some critics object that the golden rule does not give concrete guidance about what to do. Some object that the rule sets an unrealistically high standard. And some object—and this is the complaint on which we will focus here—that it sets too low a standard, making human desires the standard of moral conduct. A contemporary example of the last objection has spread like a virus: What if a sadomasochist were to do to others as he wants others to do to him? It is a scandal how rare it is to find a response to this abusive piece of sophistry. The first principle of responsible criticism is first understand, then criticize. In the West, nourished by Judaism and Christianity, the golden rule is a principle that summarizes moral tradition, "the law and the prophets"; it is not a rule that stands in isolation from tradition. The rule functions interchangeably with the law of love for the neighbor, whose universal significance took centuries to evolve. But the objection takes the rule out of every context and treats it as though it were proposed in a vacuum as a complete theory of morality. No principle of morality should be intended as a substitute for the moral intuition inherent in the human mind—no matter how much that intuition may need to be sharpened, and no matter how much the mind's moral capacity is shaped by culture and personal habit. And no principle of morality can be understood in abstraction from the heritage of moral wisdom to which every civilization contributes.

Furthermore, the golden rule is addressed to you. You are not a sadomasochist. How do you want to be treated? Confucius, Hillel, and Jesus are confronting you. Do not dodge the encounter. Philosophers are the ones who have stooped to this counterexample. Even the sadomasochist should not be such an easy target for ridicule, since he only engages in his lamentable practices with those who consent. Indeed, if such a person were to begin to apply the golden rule generally in social interactions, he might well grow in the self-respect that the rule presupposes. The counterexample, properly considered, provokes a reinterpretation, a clarification of the golden rule. The rule, to work reliably, presupposes that the agent has a normal and sympathetic regard for others' feelings and a reasonable sense of personal dignity. It is intolerable for the golden rule to be dismissed on the basis of sophistry; but it is often most helpful to respond to sophistry not by returning abuse for abuse but by spelling out the clarification that the objection requires. Many of those who use the counterexample do so with dissatisfaction, and they welcome the reply for which they had secretly hoped. The golden rule is the most widespread formula of morality in the world today, and it deserves a far better quality of attention than it has received from all but a handful of contemporary scholars.

EMPATHY AND UNDERSTANDING

One of the most fascinating topics for interdisciplinary inquiry associated with the golden rule is the practice of "putting yourself in the other person's shoes." This practice has been the object of excessive criticism and excessive esteem. The excessive criticism is that imagining oneself in another person's situation is an abstract, artificial, male, manipulative technique. The excessive esteem is the impression (which if made explicit would be quickly rejected) that imagining oneself in the other's situation unlocks new knowledge of the other and offers an unfailing guide to moral insight.

What is the value of imaginatively identifying with another person? It enables the agent to let go of a self-centered perspective—a crucial ethical advance—and it enables the person to bring to mind what he or she already knows about the other person and the situation, so as to give due weight to that information and perspective.

One reason to imagine the situation from the other's perspective is that our own immediate, intuitive grasp of a situation may not be adequate. To be sure, we need to rely every day on our intuitive sense of others. Without it, we would not have a basis of acquaintance with people at all. Moreover, once we have sharpened this intuition through imagination, education, and interaction, we continue to rely on it. Nevertheless, research shows that in surprisingly many situations we do not understand others as well as we think we do. Three professors of nursing report that even many helping professionals do not demonstrate empathy effectively.[3] In order to cultivate empathy as a skill, they developed a program for nurses in the burn unit of the hospital at Dalhousie University. The nurses learned to verbalize their intuitive grasp of the cognitive and emotional levels of what the other person was saying, and they got feedback to confirm or correct their intuition. After initial resistance to the training, the nurses developed a positive interest in the program. They learned to understand their patients and serve more effectively, and they sustained their higher levels of empathy many months after the training was over.

In short, an ideal understanding of another person requires intuition, imagination, interaction, and more, including an awareness of the history and arts of the other's tradition. The practice of imagining oneself in the other's situation is just a step, albeit an important one, in this direction.

Even an excellent understanding of another person, however, is not enough to answer ethical questions about how to interact. Empathetic understanding can lead to sympathetic behavior that might be shortsighted and harmful to the other person's long-term interests. The impulse to act on sympathy may fail to acknowledge the dignity of the other person as a rational being capable of freely making his or her own decisions. Respect for the other as an individual may fail to take adequate account of relevant aspects of the social system (such as the family, organization, or political unit) within which the interaction is taking place. Those who are indirectly affected by an action may need to be taken into account. Moreover, justice often requires interaction, so that there is not just one person imagining and deciding for everyone concerned. Thus, others whose interests are affected will have a fair opportunity to express themselves regarding the decision to be taken. Contemporary discussions of such issues are contributing to a modern, mature, expanded, and flexible interpretation of the golden rule.

REFLECTING ON HOW WE HAVE BEEN WELL TREATED

One suggestion implicit in the golden rule is to consider how you would (responsibly) want to be treated in a given situation, and it is helpful to take time for an exercise: Recall how you have been well treated in the past. Think of others who have treated you well. How did they make you feel? What was it about them and what they did that contributed to that wonderful effect? What motivated them? I do not believe we can completely answer these questions, but they are helpful in providing us with ideas about how to treat others.

This exercise also gives an occasion for us to realize that the gracious flavor of goodness that we experience when people treat us well is not something that humans simply do. Interpreting this fact of experience carries us to the limits of secular, philosophic ethics.

There is a spiritual flavor to the spontaneous generosity we experience when others treat us well, a flavor we cannot simply manufacture. The beauty of genuine goodness goes beyond the conscientious performance of duty. We begin to realize that the way we like to be treated involves a dimension that, to say the least, is not under the immediate control of the human will. The Confucian tradition of the golden rule placed particular emphasis on moving beyond conscientiousness to spontaneity.

Talking about the Spirit in a Pluralistic Environment

In the West, it is common to use the word "spiritual" to describe the flavor of gracious interaction, and the spiritual dimension of the golden rule may well be considered one of the essentials to be included in any adequate discussion. To mention spirit, however, raises a question about how fully the golden rule can be discussed in public education, since our culture is so unsettled now about how the schools should handle—or refuse to touch—religion.

In many a seminary and church-affiliated school as well as in public schools, the diversity of belief is so great that one cannot assume common ground for talking about the spirit. My practice at Kent State University is to speak of spirit while acknowledging a plurality of possible interpretations.

Beyond the Conscious Mind. Psychologists such as William James (in *Varieties of Religious Experience*) have recorded experiences in which people have solved problems and have had their lives transformed by energy and inspiration from beyond the conscious mind. Even if we regard these experiences as originating simply in the subconscious, we must acknowledge them as fact. Atheists and agnostics can speak of spirit in this sense. (Note how the popular talk of "the human spirit"—a term vaguely designating a positive attitude or a source of positive attitude—voids any religious commitments.) For some people, it is enough to connect the word "spirit" with a center of creativity associated with the right brain.

The Spirit Within. Those who have had clear experiences of "the spirit within" do not report a second personality dwelling within the human personality. The indwelling spirit, rather, is characterized as non-personal or prepersonal or transpersonal or impersonal; and this concept opens the door to interpretation from the perspective of Eastern religions (to generalize crudely).

The Spirit as the Gift of God. The spirit may also be regarded as the gift of a loving, personal God. The Hebrew scriptures speak of the image of God and of the "spirit in man" as "the candle of the Lord, searching all the inward parts" (Gen. 1:26; Prov. 20:27). Jesus taught that "the kingdom of God is within you" (Luke 17:21). The Qur'an says that God is "closer to man than his jugular vein" (Sura 50 [Qaf], section 2, verse 16).

THE GOLDEN RULE AS A SHARED PRINCIPLE IN PHILOSOPHIC AND RELIGIOUS ETHICS

Modern philosophy arose in the hope of establishing wisdom on a foundation more solid than disputed theology; and western philosophy has increasingly exiled the spiritual until recently, when multiculturalism has renewed the quest for wisdom. The demand to tear down the monopoly of the academic paradigms established by those classified as male and Eurocentric has opened the door to much that is extreme and foolish and also to much that is creative and spiritually progressive.

Looking at the worst contemporary tendencies, we could fear that our egoistic individualism, hedonistic immorality, political irresponsibility, and other follies will plunge us into a new dark age whose horrors already pervade much of the internet and the media and many homes, neighborhoods, and regions of our planet.

Looking at the best contemporary tendencies, we can also look forward to an age that is post-secular without returning to the cultural totalitarianism of the medieval church. Someday truth and beauty and goodness will prevail in our world. That will be a world in which the practice of the golden rule will flourish.

Even now, in education and society the golden rule can function as a unifier among religious and non-religious people for several reasons.

1. The golden rule is part of a non-theological philosophy of living. A person does not need to be religious in order to begin working with the golden rule and to experience the growth that such practice induces. Cooperation with the spirit is not necessarily conscious, however much prayer may illumine the situation calling for decision and action.

2. The golden rule is a principle of how everyone should relate with everyone. It makes no room for religious feelings of superiority or prejudice of any kind, including anti-religious prejudice. The rule is the most widely honored moral principle the world over, among diversely religious and non-religious groups alike.

3. The golden rule directs us away from debate and toward action, interaction, cooperation, and service. The problems facing our world are so serious that we all need to work together. The common enemy is the selfish drive to grab comfort, wealth, pleasure, and power at whatever cost to others, to future generations, and to a person's own character and soul.

4. The golden rule emphasizes what we have in common. As important as it is, this point requires clarification and qualification, to do justice to the grain of truth in the postmodern criticism that emphasizing what people have in common represses the recognition of difference, the otherness of the other. We interpret our commonalities differently (one reason that the golden rule is no panacea), although just attempting to practice the rule moves us toward the social sensitivity and moral reasoning that the best of recent philosophy promotes. Golden-rule attention to what people have in common is no excuse for disregarding the other's unique and mysteriously wonderful personality nor for disregarding differences of sex, race, class, and so on. We do not want others to disregard relevant features of who we are—but neither do we want to be treated as though some particular feature were the whole story of our identity.

A Dilemma for Religious Ethics

Of the many spiritual interpretations of the golden rule, my favorite ones are "Treat others as sons and daughters of God, as you want others to treat you," and "Treat others as God would treat them." (Note that this interpretation does not intend to justify a condescending and superior attitude, but rather proposes the same conduct that the agent would welcome from someone else in a comparable situation.) Ultimately, the golden rule is the principle of the practice of the family of God. It rests upon a prior grasp of self and others as siblings in the universal family. In order for this interpretation of the golden rule to gain recognition among ethicists, even those sympathetic to religion, an obstacle to religious ethics must be cleared away.

If someone proposes to treat someone divinely or in accord with the will of God, many philosophers reply by raising a standard dilemma: Is the act right because God wills it, or does God will it because it is right? If you say that it is right because God wills it, then you are allegedly vulnerable to the arbitrary commands of a brutal deity. If you say that God wills it because it is right, you are allegedly in no further need of God and should turn directly to the task of figuring out what is right by the standards of moral reason. If this dilemma cannot be resolved, the game is over for religious ethics and the technical sophistication of secular ethics will be the best we have to offer.

This alleged dilemma falsifies the experience of seeking and living the will of God. First of all, the God whom we find, by the aid of revelation, in our experience of prayer and worship is brimming with goodness and overflowing with love, a God of sovereign wisdom and a giver of insight. Therefore the problem about a brutal deity manifests the same sophistry that assails the golden rule, and the objection is valid only against a philosopher's construct, a theory that would reduce the adventure of seeking for God and God's way into a simplistic formula. The benefit of considering the objection, however, is to recall that where traditional scriptures imply brutality in their concept of God, those passages must be rejected by morally and spiritually sensitive persons.

The second problem, about the relevance of God to moral inquiry, requires a number of points in response. Modern moral reason presupposes the equal dignity of each person as a (potentially) rational agent, but when that assumption is shaken, it reveals its need of a religious basis: the equal spiritual dignity of the sons and daughters of the Creator, the universal Father. Moral reason considers principles, but principles do not always suffice to indicate the best and right way to proceed. Moral reason considers situational details and the history of practices and relationships, but such information does not always suffice. So a human being who has exhausted the human capacity for moral inquiry has an understandable desire to reach for a source of superhuman insight. Some ethical theories imagine an Ideal Observer with complete information and perfect sympathy with everyone affected by the action under consideration. Moreover, even when the right action has been found, the gracious way to perform that course of action requires spiritual spontaneity. Some ethical theories are part of a larger system of philosophy or theology in which the reality of God is affirmed. Then prayer makes sense, and the labor of moral reason can become a phase of a responsible prayer process. Finally, if the highest goal of human character achievement is to become like God, then the more we know of God the more we can participate in this amazing growth project whose initial phase we know as life on planet earth.

Ethics at its fullest, I believe, is religious ethics, the adventure of seeking, finding, choosing, and doing the will of God. When the agony of a hard decision is upon us, it is no simple matter to find the will of God. Paying attention to great commandments and ethical principles, exploring the situation, conversing with morally wise persons, studying philosophy, literature, and the biographies of those who manifest the grandeur of genuine character achievement—all these can help. In the end, however, these phases of inquiry are preliminary; they do not make the decision for us; they do not adequately illumine our path. Rather, we gradually learn to cooperate with a wisdom beyond our ken, to enter, by our decisions, into a process which we cannot govern, although we may have responsibility for mastering ourselves or for providing leadership or even for prevailing in some regard. Those who reject religion may interpret the inner source of wisdom, creativity, inspiration, joy and peace as part of human nature, but their techniques of tapping that source will fall short of the relational dynamism of religious faith. Only religious living brings the golden rule to fruition.

Conclusion

To recapitulate, education promotes not only success but growth as well. Growth involves service, and service involves the practice of the golden rule. The principle, Do to others as you want others to do to you, deserves study and application throughout our educational system, on moral and religious grounds.

NOTES

1. I present a fuller account of these stories in *The Golden Rule* (New York: Oxford University Press, 1996). I am indebted to Greensboro College for the opportunity to develop these ideas further in the 1997 Jean Fortner Ward Lecture.
2. See Kant's notorious critique of the golden rule in his footnote at Ak. 430 of the *Grounding*.
3. See "Learning to use empathy" by three professors of nursing at Dalhousie University, Jean R. Hughes, E. Joyce Carver, and Ruth C. MacKay in Ruth C. MacKay, Jean R. Hughes, and E. Joyce Carver, eds., *Empathy and the Helping Relationship* (New York: Springer, 1990). For a discussion of the problem of empathic error, see *The Golden Rule*, 115-117.

QUESTIONS FOR DISCUSSION

1. Do those in what have traditionally been considered helping professions have an advantage in practicing and fulfilling the Golden Rule? Why or why not?

2. Have you tried to place yourself in someone else's position? Was this difficult? Why or why not?

3. Under what circumstances is one propelled into putting him or herself in another person's situation?

4. What role does reflection play in practicing the Golden Rule?

5. When is sympathy harmful? Why? How?

6. How can we assist others in developing and expressing their views where issues of justice are concerned?

7. What would a modern classroom guided by the Golden Rule be like?

8. What do teachers, parents, and leaders need to know about the Golden Rule in order to be ethically educated?

9. Since the Golden Rule cannot be reduced to a simplistic formula, how can adults communicate these ideals to the young?

10. How is acting with the knowledge that we are children of God different from acting with the knowledge that we are rational moral agents? What are the consequences of these differences?

CHRISTIAN ETHICS
CHRIST, COVENANT, CREATION

Charles S. McCoy

ABSTRACT

Ethics as reflection on the moral significance of action takes place in all human communities and relies on some tradition of faith. Similar in derivation, morality and ethics should be distinguished, morality meaning customary standards of behavior and ethics referring to critical reflection about morals. Two problems plague ethics today: rationalism focused on concepts rather than on moral action and individualism that ignores organizational action. Christian ethics is best understood by means of three themes: first, the center of Christian faith and ethics in Jesus Christ and his new commandment of love; second, the communal character of ethics revealed in God's covenant in the Old and New Testaments; third, creation in God, making clear the comprehensiveness of Christian faith and ethics; the inclusiveness of the commandment of love; and the resources available for guiding moral choice and action. Federal ethics, which permeates Western societies, emphasizes virtue as social achievement. Finally, Christian faith and ethics relies on the sovereignty of God.

G. K. Chesterton tells a story about a man who could shoot his grandmother at 500 yards. We would have no difficulty, Chesterton readily affirms, in calling him a "good shot," but might have reservations about calling him a "good person." There is no doubt that his technical ability is excellent; his moral goodness is questionable. An example in recent history of a similar combination is Adolf Hitler, who, according to a biographer, Alan Bullock, was an amazingly quick study when it came to grasping data of a technical nature but verged on being tone deaf when it came to moral values.

Institutions of higher education are usually better about training people to be good shots than to be good persons, better at educating students in technical know-how than preparing them to engage in ethical reflection or to participate in shaping society and its multiple organizations in moral directions. By no means is that to say that technical skill is not involved in ethics. A company building a bridge and the people working for it ought to have the technical skills, the resources needed to complete the project, and the ability to carry it through, as well as moral responsibility and ethical insight. The entire curriculum of colleges and universities contributes these multiple factors that are essential for building a good bridge, one that will be capable of carrying the intended traffic across the river or chasm with effectiveness and safety for many years. Ethical reflection should combine commitment to moral values, technical expertise, and effective power in human action, whether for individuals or social groups. To unite these three components, Christian ethics draws on the biblical Christian heritage of faith that pervades Western culture. Available in that heritage are the purposes, rules, and criteria of responsibility found in all academic disciplines and human experience, as well as in the Bible and theology. These resources guide the actions of organizations and persons related to the varied communities of Christian faith.

THE MEANING OF ETHICS

Ethics can be understood most comprehensively as reflection within community on the moral significance of human action. As such it takes place in every human tradition and community—Hindu, Jewish, Confucian, Buddhist, Christian, and Moslem; communist, socialist, and capitalist; cultural, national, and ethnic; corporate, professional, and activist. Ethical reflection goes on in organized groups as well as among individuals. It permeates human life, just as do religion, economics, politics, sexuality, education, and family or tribe. Ethics involves goals and purposes, codes of conduct and laws, life styles, and the discernment of appropriate action in particular social locations. Ethics can be discerned in the enveloping action of a literary work, in the presuppositions and methods of social scientists, and in the network of commitments to be found in communities of physical scientists. Ethics takes groups and individuals believe has enduring reality, meaning, and value, and is reflected in *action* systems.

Some would argue that ethics is completely relative because it differs from one community to another, while others affirm that it is absolute because there are ethical principles that all communities agree upon. Neither view can withstand careful examination. To adopt the first view requires absolutizing relativism, a contradiction unacceptable to those who take reason seriously. Affirming the second view overlooks the differing interpretations of principles within different communities, even though they are phrased in similar ways. Both relativism and absolutism in ethics involve what can be called "the fallacy of dichotomous thinking," the error of beginning with polar opposites, then affirming one to the exclusion of the other (absolute or relative in this case; other examples of dichotomies often found in Western thought are objective or subjective, mental or physical, noumenal or phenomenal, individual or community, etc.). A dichotomy is useful only where there is agreement on the framework for judging, e.g., as in ordinary arithmetic where the answer to a problem can be said to be right or wrong, or in sectarian enclaves of a religious or academic type in which the participants share similar dogmatic convictions. Dichotomous thinking runs roughshod over the ambiguities of the human situation.

Though many hope that ethics will disclose a realm of clear, easily perceived right and wrong, moral experience retains considerable ambiguity, especially across cultures but also within communities considered to possess a general homogeneity. Ethical reflection does, however, enable humans to see choices more clearly. Through the tangled environment of values, moral directives, and behavioral valences in which humanity is immersed from womb to tomb, ethics provides guidance for action.

Ethics and morality are closely related and, though sometimes identified, must be distinguished. The term "ethics" derives from the Greek *ēthikē*, and "moral" derives from the Latin *mos, mores* (pl.). In their original meaning in Hellenic and Graeco-Roman cultures, both words mean approximately the same thing—customs, usual ways of acting, conventional behavior, or character. Over the centuries, however, their meanings have diverged. Morals or morality have retained a meaning closer to that to be found in ancient cultures. Ethics has taken on a meaning involving critical reflection about morality and resources for combining and modifying conventional directives for behavior. In similar fashion, Christian ethics and Christian morality must be distinguished. Indeed, Jesus Christ as the focus of Christian faith provides a model for the distinction between ethics and morality and enunciates a new basis of ethical reflection—the commandment of love—as the central criterion for re-evaluation and modification of the morality inherited from the past.

THE PLIGHT OF ETHICS

Ethics today has serious internal problems that render it ill-equipped to wrestle with the challenging moral issues of our time, organizational or individual. The most important and debilitating of these problems are rationalism and individualism.

In a book first published in 1960 Mary Warnock has this to say in criticism of academic ethics in England:

> One of the consequences of treating ethics as the analysis of ethical language is, as I have suggested earlier, that it leads to the increasing triviality of the subject ... One aspect of this trivializing of the subject is the refusal of moral philosophers in England to commit themselves to any moral opinions.[1]

The same criticism can be leveled at ethics in America, in part because scholars in this country chose to follow the flawed example of their English counterparts. Philosophical ethics almost trivialized itself out of existence but made a recovery in the 1970's by entering the field of business ethics. Many even in Christian ethics followed the same path into a wasteland of rationalism as they tried to reduce ethics to ethical theory. Warnock explains why theory alone is inadequate in ethics:

> In ethics, alone among the branches of philosophical study, the subject matter is not so much the categories which we use to describe or to learn about the world, as our own impact upon the world, our relation to other people and our attitude to our situation and our life. We do need to categorize and to describe, even in the sphere of morals, but we should still exist as moral agents even if we seldom did so; and therefore the subject matter of ethics would still exist.[2]

Though I agree with Warnock's criticism of ethics, it seems possible that the same issue can be raised about other branches of philosophy. The primary subject matter is not the rational categories used to understand the world but rather the world that scholars are seeking to describe and learn about. Indeed, the field of natural philosophy disappeared a few centuries ago because it developed its own categories about nature and then expected nature to obey the rational deductions of the philosophers! The rise of modern science effectively displaced natural philosophy by giving primary attention to nature and continually reshaping scientific categories to fit what was observed. Ethics, to the extent that it limits its attention to ethical theory, finds itself in a situation similar to that of natural philosophy four centuries ago—increasingly trivial and obsolescent. In ethics, reason is needed as a tool, but reason itself is not the focus of study. Moral choice and action in human communities, as well as ethical categories, must be adjusted and reshaped to fit the changing environment of issues and values.

The individualism that became increasingly prominent in ethics during the twentieth century is a second problem. This development is puzzling, for it represents a radical departure from the long tradition of Western communal ethics stretching back through Karl Marx and Adam Smith, through the leaders of Reformation and medieval thought, to ancient sources in Augustine, Aristotle, Plato, and the Hebrew prophets. Ethics in this heritage is applicable to the collective dimensions of human action, not only to individual behavior. "Thus says the Lord," Amos proclaims,

> for three transgressions of Damascus and for four ... . for three transgressions of Gaza and for four ... . for three transgressions of Tyre and for four ... . for three transgressions of Edom and for four ... . for three transgressions of the Ammonites and for four ... . for three transgressions of Moab and for four ... . for three transgressions of Judah and for four ... . for three transgressions of Israel and for four, I will not revoke the punishment; because they sell the righteous for silver, and the needy for a pair of sandals—they who trample the head of the poor into the dust of the earth, and push the afflicted out of the way. (Amos 1:3; 1:6; 1:9; 1:11; 1:13; 2:1; 2:4; 2:6-7)

Isaiah, Jeremiah, and other Hebrew prophets follow suit in declaring God's judgment upon both community and individuals. Plato in *The Republic* insists that justice cannot be achieved in individual souls apart from justice in society, and justice in society cannot be developed apart from justice in individuals. Individual and society are knit together. In Aristotle and Augustine, ethics is individual, social, and political. Most thinkers of the Western tradition concur. Johannes Althusius, the first to formulate a federal political philosophy, speaks of humans as "symbiotes" rather than individuals.[3] Only as academic disciplines became separate and increasingly isolated from one another in the twentieth century has ethics all too often come to interpret human action only as individual. For ethics to be understood with appropriate wholeness, the entire spectrum of disciplines must be reconnected with one another and with human experience in community.

The individualistic focus of ethics creates serious difficulties today because we live in a world in which organizations have great power. Governments and their multiplying agencies, business corporations, political parties, labor unions, educational institutions, religious groups, the legal and the medical professions—all have, as organizations, great influence on society, on the conditions of human existence, and on the actions of individuals in the organizations. The morality of organizations poses issues of urgency and difficulty for humanity in the contemporary world—urgent because the welfare of the earth and its inhabitants depends upon the values guiding the actions of organizations; difficult because organizations have become large and complex. The plight of ethics has been compounded as ethics has focused more and more on theory and individual morality, while social scientists who seek to understand organizations have tried to be "value-free" in their research and avoid involvement with ethics.

Individualism has infected Christian ethics as well as philosophical ethics, though not in quite so virulent a form. Many leaders within the Christian community, both scholars and church officials, have continued to be concerned about the ethics of organizations and their impact on social justice, though their proposals for solutions have tended for the most part to remain rooted in individualism.[4]

On the other hand, the rise of protest movements against injustice and discrimination has helped to raise issues about the ethics of organizations. As protests have been successful, the need to move from protest to policy has underscored the need to move beyond individualism. In the 1970's, considerable progress was made toward the re-invention of the field of organizational ethics, to relate ethics again to the social and natural sciences, and to involve ethics directly with the experience of concerned people working in centers of social power and change. From these expanded experiences and developments, it has become clear that Christian ethics must learn not only to draw deeply on its resources in the Bible and in the Christian heritage, but also to discover ways to absorb lessons from other traditions and cultures.

UNDERSTANDING CHRISTIAN ETHICS

At one point in *Alice in Wonderland,* Alice is lost and requests assistance from the Cheshire Cat. "Would you tell me, please, which way I ought to go from here?"

"That depends a good deal on where you want to get to," the cat quite sensibly replies.

"I don't much care where," says Alice.

"Then," concludes the Cheshire Cat, "it doesn't matter which way you go."

Unless we have commitments as to destination, directives about travel will be of no use to us. In this sense, ethics and morals are dependent upon faith, i.e., upon what a person or a community believes in as real, meaningful, and valuable. This faith may derive from one of the major religious communities of the world, each of which has ethics and morals based upon the ultimate commitments of that community; or faith may be in reason, in one's nation, in humanity, or in communism.

In the ancient world of the Bible and Hellenic society, objects of devotion providing guidance for living were designated as deities. The cultural triumph of Jewish and Christian faith in Western society resulted in giving the name God only to the deity of the biblical tradition; the other gods described and named in the Bible are first reduced to the status of idols and then eliminated from discussions of religion and ethics. These other objects of devotion are still present in new forms, but today are relegated to the catch-all category of the "secular." Theologians as well as others have divided the world into "believers" and "non-believers." Pollsters ask, "Do you believe in God?" As a result, we are left with the problem: what do the unbelievers believe? And some of us think a more revealing question to ask the public is: "What god or gods do you believe in?" A more inclusive notion of deity would also have made it easier for Western scholars in the study of religion and ethics to recognize that members of other than Western religions were not non-believers and were not without traditions of ethical reflection.

Christian ethics emerges from the context of faith within the Christian community. It draws its principles and criteria for ethical reflection from the Bible, the Christian tradition, and the experience of Christians in each contemporary period. Christian ethics makes use of reason but is not governed by it as is philosophical ethics. Contemporary experience to be drawn upon includes the spectrum of disciplines in higher education and the plurality of perspectives and knowledge present in global society.

With this perspective on the problems and possibilities of Christian ethics, we can turn our attention directly to an understanding of ethical reflection within the Christian community of faith. Three themes provide the basic pattern of Christian ethics: Jesus Christ, God's covenant, and creation in God.

JESUS CHRIST

The center of Christian faith and ethics is Jesus Christ. Sources for understanding this focus of faith are the Gospels, providing first-hand accounts by his followers of his life and teachings, crucifixion, and resurrection, assembled later by the emerging Christian community; the Old Testament, the Scriptures of the Hebrew tradition within which Jesus lived and from which Christianity came; the early proclamations of the meaning of Jesus Christ as provided in the New Testament writings; and the experience of Christians within the Christian heritage over two millennia.

When Christians confess their faith, it is not primarily in books of theology or philosophy but rather by telling the story of Jesus Christ—his life in an outlying Jewish province of the Roman Empire, his death on a cross at the hands of Roman soldiers, and his resurrection as his followers experienced and reported it. In the vivid words of Paul, the great messenger of this Gospel that endured the persecution of Rome and eventually conquered the Empire:

> Now I want you to remember, my brothers and sisters, the Good News that I preached to you, that you accepted as your own, and in which your faith is firmly rooted. That is the Good News through which you are saved, if you hold that message firmly in memory—unless your believing was not real. For I passed on to you as of first importance that which in turn I had accepted: that Christ died for our sins as Scripture tells us; that Christ was buried and raised to life again also according to Scripture; and that Peter saw him alive and then also all the apostles, and later more than five hundred disciples, most of whom are still alive. After that he appeared to James and again to the apostles. And finally, he appeared to me, and I experienced the strange power of new birth. (1 Cor. 15:1-8)

Christian faith has a "storied," historical quality that provides its distinctive core. "The preaching of the early Christian church," writes H. Richard Niebuhr, who perceived this basic nature of Christianity long before "story" became a theological fad,

> was not an argument for the existence of God nor an admonition to follow the dictates of some common human conscience ... . It was primarily a simple recital of the great events connected with the historical appearance of Jesus Christ and a confession of what had happened to the community of disciples.[5]

Niebuhr also saw clearly that Christian faith comes to us, not when we merely hear the story, but rather when it becomes "the story of our life," our story, our very own story, when we have internalized it so it is the way we understand ourselves, our companions on this journey in time, and the world in which we live. The story of our life through Jesus Christ shapes Christian faith and ethics. Our storied existence, our participation in the story, tells us what is real, what is meaningful, and what is of value.

The life and teachings of Jesus provide the core of Christian ethics because he is believed in as Christ, the Messiah, the anointed of God. The Messiah is anticipated throughout the Old Testament as divinely designated to be prophet, priest, and leader of God's people. To these roles Christian faith adds belief in Jesus Christ as revelation and manifestation of God.

The basis of Jesus' ethic is God's love for us, a love that calls us to respond in love to God and neighbor. As the Gospel of John tells us: "For God loved the world so much as to offer God's son, that those who believe in him may have eternal life" (John 3:16). God's love embraces the entire world. Before God no one is an alien—unless they alienate themselves. When a lawyer asks Jesus what he must do to inherit eternal life, Jesus elicits the answer of response to God's love: "You shall love the Lord your God with all your heart, and with all your soul, and with all your strength, and with all your mind; and your neighbor as yourself." Jesus replies: "You have answered correctly" (Luke 10:25-28). In John, Jesus repeats this injunction in slightly different form: "A new commandment I give you, that you love one another just as I have loved you" (John 13:34). In the passage on the judgment of the nations in Matthew, Jesus takes the commandment further and affirms that, in loving neighbors by feeding the hungry, providing something to drink for the thirsty, welcoming strangers, giving clothing to the naked, caring for the sick, or visiting those in prison, we are responding with love to God (Matt. 25:31-46). In many parables and actions of healing, and above all in the crucifixion and resurrection, Jesus embodies God's love for the world and the call to respond with love toward God and neighbor.

The new commandment of love given by Jesus calls humans to levels of response beyond laws and rules, even to actions that Reinhold Niebuhr labels an "impossible possibility."[6] Jesus' call to love does not, however, abolish law but rather fulfills law and is its purpose (Matt. 5:17 and Rom. 10:4). The command of love also provides a criterion for evaluating the moral directives inherited from the past—and for changing them. Jesus provides the model for continuing re-evaluation of tradition; this process of loyalty to tradition and modification of it is essential to Christian ethical reflection as humans move toward completion and fulfillment in God (see Matt. 5:21-48).

The commandment of love includes from the Hebrew heritage the call of God to justice and liberation. Emerging throughout Jesus' teaching and actions, these prophetic themes are stated most clearly in the messianic proclamation of his mission when he speaks in the synagogue at Nazareth:

> When he arrived in Nazareth, where he had been brought up, he went as was his custom to the synagogue on the Sabbath. There he stood up to read from the scroll of the prophet Isaiah that had been handed him. He unrolled it and found the passage where it was written—
>
> > The Spirit of the Lord is upon me,
> > because he has anointed me
> > to bring good news to the poor.
> > He has sent me to proclaim
> > release to the captives
> > and recovery of sight to the blind,
> > to set at liberty those who are oppressed,
> > and to proclaim the presence of
> > God's loving-kindness.
>
> He then rolled up the scroll, returned it to the attendant, and sat down. The eyes of everyone in the synagogue were focused on him. And he said to them, "Today this scripture is being fulfilled in our presence." (Luke 4:16-21)

As this account emphasizes, Jesus Christ as the center of the Christian story points beyond himself to the wider context of Christianity: to the history of Hebrew faith in the Old Testament, where the messianic character of Jesus' message and the resources for ethics are expanded; to the New Testament, as the Christian church emerges and spreads in the wake of the resurrection; to the heritage of Christian experience over two millennia; and to God as the ultimate and immediate context of humanity and the world.

GOD'S COVENANT

Just as Jesus Christ is the center, so God's covenant with the world and with humanity underscores the communal character of Christian faith and ethics. The theme of God's covenant provides perspective on this larger setting of Christian faith and ethics. Christianity is about God's relationship to humanity through community, history, and creation. The Bible from beginning to end describes this relation as covenantal, a term that can also be used to characterize both primitive and developed societies as well as the natural world.

The idea of covenant permeates both the Old and New Testaments. Indeed, the word "testament" comes from the Latin *testamentum*, the term used in the Vulgate (Latin Bible) to translate the Hebrew $b^e rîth$, meaning covenant. The Old Testament scholar, Walther Eichrodt, focuses his three-volume *Theologie des alten Testaments* on the covenant and on Yahweh as the Covenant God. The covenant, says Eichrodt, is "the critical term for Israelite thought" and "the basic principle of the relationship to God."[7] Other concepts important for ethics in the Old Testament must be understood within God's covenant. For example, *mishpāt* means justice, not in some general sense, but covenant-justice; *hesed* is covenant loving-kindness; and Hebrew history has its focus in Yahweh's covenant faithfulness and steadfastness.[8] Martin Buber asserts that it is impossible to grasp the inner coherence of the faith of Israel without understanding the covenant.[9] The Hebrew nation is founded on the covenant made at Sinai (Exod. 19:5; 24:7ff.) after the liberation from bondage in Egypt, events that come to define the meaning of Hebrew history and identity. The covenant is understood as made by God in the creation of the entire natural order (Jer. 33:20-25), broken from the human side by Adam (Hos. 6:7) but upheld and renewed by God with Noah (Gen. 9:8ff.), with Abraham (Gen. 15:17f.; 17:7), and with Jacob (Gen. 28:18ff.; 35:9ff.). Bernard Anderson writes: "The peculiar nature of the Hebrew community is expressed in the covenant relationship between Yahweh and the people of Israel, and the Laws and institutions by which this relationship is expressed is... the core of the life of this people."[10]

The Hebrew prophets speak within this covenantal context, calling a faithless Israel back to God, the Faithful One. Jeremiah declares a new covenant (Jer. 31:33ff.) that Jesus affirms: "This cup which is poured out for you is the new covenant in my blood" (Luke 22:20), a theme taken up again and again throughout the New Testament.

In biblical perspective, covenant means an unconditional agreement of community, friendship, peace, and justice, with dimensions of both faith and ethics. Covenant can be contrasted with what is usually called a contract, which involves a conditional agreement where the obligation of either party depends upon performance of certain actions by the other. Parties to a covenant are committed to one another whether there is performance or not. Covenant is gift and grace, a means for overcoming enmity, alienation, and conflict, as when Jonathan and David made a covenant, and "the soul of Jonathan was knit to the soul of David" (1 Sam. 18:1). Covenant points back to the creation by God the Faithful One and forward through the promise in the messianic tradition to fulfillment and consummation in God.

The promise of community within God's covenant extends the theme of the inclusive love of God found in the Gospels. There is no special approval of the rich and successful as was implied in some versions of Calvinism, nor an option for the poor, as some liberation theologians suggest. Rain falls on the just and unjust. The plumb line of justice judges individuals and nations, rich and poor. The love of God in Jesus Christ reaches out to Zaccheus and Nicodemus, to the Gerasene demoniac and the woman at the well of Samaria, to the rich ruler as well as to the poor, the oppressed, and the sick. Like a magnetic field exercising power over all, the covenant of God in community calls all humans to respond to God's justice and love within and through each particular social location and relation.

In the light of the biblical message of Jesus Christ and God's covenant, it is strange to discover some church leaders today telling Christians they are "resident aliens." Just the opposite teaching is found in the Bible. As we read in Ephesians:

> remember that once you were without Christ, being aliens from the community of Israel, and strangers to the covenants of promise, living in the world without hope and without God. But now in Christ Jesus you who then were far off have been brought near by the blood of Jesus Christ. For he is our peace.... So Jesus Christ came and brought peace to you who were far off and peace to those already near; for through him both have access through one Spirit to God. Now you are no longer strangers and aliens, but you are citizens, just as are saints and members of the household of God, founded on the apostles and prophets with Jesus Christ as the cornerstone. (Eph. 2:12-14, 17-21)

In Egypt, the Israelites were indeed resident aliens, but God delivered them from bondage, made covenant with them, and led them into a homeland. Even when the Babylonian exiles were in a political sense resident aliens, God directs them through Jeremiah to treat the land of exile as a homeland:

> Thus says the Lord of hosts, the God of Israel, to all the exiles whom I have sent into exile from Jerusalem to Babylon: Build houses and live in them; plant gardens and eat their produce. Take wives and have sons and daughters; take wives for your sons, and give your daughters in marriage, that they in turn may have sons and daughters; increase there as a people rather than decrease. And seek the welfare of the city wherein I have sent you into exile, and pray to God on its behalf, for in its welfare you will find your welfare. (Jer. 29:4-7)

In no way are Christians resident aliens in this world that God created and enters in Jesus Christ to liberate and redeem. When humans rebel against God, they alienate themselves from God, from their fellow human beings, and from their own being. Then indeed they are resident aliens in the world, as were the

Israelites in Egypt. But God is the Faithful One. The covenant of God and God's love for the world remain. As Jesus Christ overcomes estrangement, we can discover that we are no longer strangers and aliens in a strange land, but residents and citizens of the homeland in which we were created by God. Prodigal sons and daughters, resident aliens in a far country, we may discover ourselves to be, but the home we left is still there, and a welcome awaits us where we are neither strangers nor aliens. Christian ethics emerges from the awareness that we are children of God, called to seek the welfare of all within our homeland.

CREATION IN GOD

"How can Christianity call itself catholic," asks Simone Weil, "if the universe itself is left out?"[11] The affirmation of God as creator opens the way to include the creation, but the significance of the entire world of nature for Christian faith and ethics is seldom explored.

The center of Christian faith and ethics is Jesus Christ. The communal nature of our faith and ethics is revealed in God's covenant as it unfolds in the Old and New Covenants. And the understanding of the creation of the world in God makes clear the comprehensiveness and inclusiveness, beyond thought and imagination, of that which Christians believe and the resources available as we reflect on our moral choices and actions.

As we explore the implications of creation in Christian faith, we find ourselves on a journey with surprising vistas and a destination glimpsed only in faith. It is one thing to affirm in faith that God created this world of unfolding complexity and mystery. It is quite another to affirm that we glimpse the meaning at the heart of this mystery. That, however, is what the Prologue to the Gospel of John tells us. What does it mean? What are its implications?

The Greek word *logos* is almost universally translated into modern languages as "Word," or its cognate (e.g., *Wort* in German, *parole* in French). James Moffatt in his version leaves it as "Logos."[12] The explanation of the meaning of "Word" has caused commentators continuing difficulty. Most often they resort to the meaning of *logos* in Greek thought, where it appears in both Hellenic and Hellenistic writings. It seems highly dubious, however, that the writer of the fourth Gospel was attempting to convey Greek philosophy to his readers. The great German poet Goethe in Faust protests strongly against the use of *Wort* as impossible. He proposes *Sinn* (meaning or mind) as a more acceptable choice but turns finally to *Akt* (action) as better if one is to speak of it as the basis of creation. Goethe has a point: creation involves power, not merely meaning or voice. Rather than teaching Christians Greek thought, John was clearly trying to convey the Hebraic background of Christianity to a Christian community immersed in Greek culture. Building on Goethe's suggestion and remembering that the Septuagint translators used *logos* to render the Hebrew *dābār*, a more adequate translation into English would be "faithful action." Such a rendering is in keeping with the covenantal tradition and its meaning for Jesus Christ in the New Testament:

> In the beginning was the Faithful Action. The Faithful Action was with God, and the Faithful Action was God. In the very beginning the Faithful Action was with God. All things that exist came into being through the Faithful Action, and apart from the Faithful Action of God not a single thing exists. In God's Faithful Action is life, and this life provides light for all humanity. This light shines in the midst of darkness, and the darkness is unable to destroy it... .
>
> The Faithful Action was already in the world, for the world existed through the Faithful Action, yet the world did not recognize him. He entered his own homeland, but his own kin did not accept him. But to all who did accept him, who recognize their reliance upon him, he confers the right to become children of God, who know they owe their being to God rather than to human blood or the impulse of human flesh.
>
> So the Faithful Action has become flesh and has made his home with us. We have beheld his glory, the glory that a child shares with his parent, and have seen him full of grace and reality... . While the Law was given through Moses, grace and reality are ours through Jesus Christ. No person has ever seen God, but God has revealed the Divine Self only in this One who is at one with the Creator (John 1:1-5, 10-14, 17-18, my translation).

That to which we respond in every human encounter, in the entire range of human experience, is the Faithful One, the God of covenant glimpsed in Jesus Christ. The reliance by physical scientists and all scholarship on the consistency of the universe through time past and time future as well as into the farthest reaches of the cosmos reflects response to this Faithful One. This reality reveals moral no less than physical reliability, a consistency reflected in human communities in all cultures and social locations.

In speaking of Brother Sun and Sister Moon, Francis of Assisi acknowledges the natural world as part of God's covenanted order. We are responding to God's faithfulness and love as we respond to the environment that God loves and through which God expresses love for humanity. In their creation by God, humans near and far are our sisters and brothers in Jesus Christ. Whether they recognize it or not, Christian faith and ethics call us to respond to God's faithful action in every human life.

Christians can learn about the Faithful One wherever humans explore the creation. In the Christian heritage, human experience of God in other religions, in all academic disciplines, in the complexity of ordinary relationships, and in emerging investigations of the macro-cosmos and micro-cosmos, have meaning for faith and ethics. Our understanding of Jesus Christ is deepened, not diluted, by expanding our Christian faith and ethics to include the insights of other cultures and the full range of human learning in all its dimensions. *Your God is Too Small*, J. B. Phillips reminds us, helping us to see Christianity more as adventure into an alluring mystery than a list of settled dogmas. Dwelling in the biblical story of Jesus Christ challenges us to break out into increasingly more inclusive understandings of God's love and justice. Michael Polanyi suggests, Christianity sustains "an eternal, never to be consummated hunch: a heuristic vision which is accepted for the sake of its unresolvable tension."[13]

VIRTUE AS SOCIAL ACHIEVEMENT

In *The Republic* (359d-360d), Plato tells the story of Gyges, a shepherd in Lydia, who found a gold ring, which he discovered had magical powers. While attending the customary assembly of shepherds to make their usual monthly report to the king, who owned the flocks, he noticed that when he turned the collet of the ring inward, he became invisible, and when he turned it outward, he was again visible. Upon making this discovery, Gyges arranged to be one of the messengers who went to the palace to report to the king. When he arrived, he made himself invisible, seduced the queen, with her aid killed the king, and became king.

Plato ponders the meaning of the story. Is anyone so committed to ethical living that he would persevere in justice if he possessed such a ring? Plato doubts that a person could be found with so firm a character, and if there were such a person, he would be regarded by others as a fool. Human nature, in Plato's view, is neither completely good nor totally evil. Virtuous behavior in individuals needs the re-enforcement of visibility in a social context; standards of morality can be ignored if one is invisible. To the extent that it can be achieved among humans, virtue is a hard-won social achievement, not something that inheres in individual character alone.

The biblical view of ethics, understood through Jesus Christ, covenant, and creation, is similar to Plato's. Christian ethics emerges in the community of faith in Christ, shaped by the covenant of God, and rooted in God's faithful action in creation.

Even Reinhold Niebuhr, who had massive impact on political thought and governmental policy in America during the middle years of the twentieth century, became entangled in ethical individualism. In *Moral Man and Immoral Society*, he says that "a sharp distinction must be drawn between the moral and social behavior of individuals and of social groups." Though he admits that the title of his book makes the distinction in a way that is too unqualified, he still maintains that individuals "may be moral in the sense that they are able to consider interests other than their own in determining problems of conduct," while in "every human group there is less reason to guide and check impulse, less capacity for self-transcendence, less ability to comprehend the needs of others and therefore more unrestrained egoism than the individuals, who compose the group, reveal in their personal relationships."[14]

Perhaps Niebuhr's own social background led him to give individuals too much exemption from sin and to forget the symbiotic relation of individual and society. The experiences of committed southerners who gave birth in the 1930's and 1940's to the civil rights movement of the 1950's and 1960's might lead them to the reverse of Niebuhr's view; they might think it more accurate to speak of "immoral man and moral society." Only by appealing beyond the unjust actions of individual southerners against Black Americans to the heritage of justice and freedom built into American society was it possible for the civil rights movement to achieve significant success. The advances in justice produced by the civil rights movement illustrate virtue as a *social*, not just an individual achievement.

Christian ethics must avoid one-sided simplifications. It is neither "moral man and immoral society" nor "immoral man and moral society." Individuals and society are too closely interrelated for either to be correct. Societies do not exist without individual members, and persons as individuals are constituted through their participation in society. To put it in biblical terms, we are created and exist within God's covenant. Ethical reflection in the Christian tradition must be concerned with the moral significance of actions by both individuals and social groups.

ETHICS AS FEDERAL

The most pervasive form of ethics operative in Western societies is federal ethics, so named because the word "federal" derives from the Latin *foedus*, which means covenant. Though most scholars in ethics give it little attention, federal ethics has exercised growing influence in recent centuries as political and economic power has moved from crown to people. Emerging from such covenanted groups as the Hanseatic League and the Swiss Confederation, federal thought was shaped by the Reformation's recovery of the Bible with its emphasis on covenants. In subsequent centuries, federal theology and ethics together with federal political and economic patterns have permeated Western societies and are spreading around the world.[15]

The clearest example of federal ethics is the United States, with its federal constitution, its federal structures in political order, economics, and religion, and its federal array of voluntary activity. The federal ideas brought by early colonists from Europe took root and assumed a distinctively American shape during the colonial period of 170 years as the British colonies developed their own traditions. With the American Revolution the separate states organized themselves around federal constitutions and an emerging national federal order. This process reached its culmination in the Federal Constitution produced by the Philadelphia Convention in 1787 and ratified by the states the following year.

The basic covenant of American society is the Preamble to the Constitution. In the Bill of Rights, religious faith is liberated from dogmatic creeds established by government and turned over to communities of covenanted believers. Though many church officials warned that faith in general and Christian faith in particular would be killed by disestablishment, quite the opposite has actually occurred. The churches have flourished and become creative and influential centers of ethical reflection and guidance for the society. Even more, the federal pattern has permitted and encouraged the proliferation of voluntary societies, from garden clubs to social action groups, that nurture a wide spectrum of interests and help the nation meet new challenges and continuing change.

In *The Federalist*, a series of papers designed to promote the ratification of the Federal Constitution, James Madison, a key figure at the Constitutional Convention, explains the federal ethics embodied in the Constitution: "What is government itself but the greatest of all reflections on human nature? If men were angels, no government would be necessary."[16] Since they are not angels, they develop factions, groups "united and actuated by some common impulse of passion, or of interest, adverse to the rights of other citizens, or to the permanent and aggregate interests of the community... . The latent causes of faction are sown in the nature of man... . the *causes* of faction cannot be removed [without destroying liberty] so relief is only to be sought in the means of controlling its *effects*" (No. 10). "Ambition must be made to counteract ambition... . This policy of supplying by opposite and rival interests, the defect of better motives, might be traced through the whole system of human affairs, private as well as public.... the constant aim is to divide and arrange the several offices in such a manner as that each may be a check on the other" (No. 51). As in religion, the rights of all are rendered more secure by a plurality of sects checking one another, so in government, "the security for civil rights.... consists in the multiplicity of interests" checking one another. Justice and the common good, as well as securing liberty and civil rights, are the aims of government, best approached "by a judicious modification and mixture of the *federal principle*" (No. 51).

Virtue in society cannot be achieved by relying upon virtuous individuals. On this the Bible, Plato, and Madison would agree. Instead, virtue, to the extent it can exist among humans, remains a hard-won social achievement, made possible by checks and balances among diverse groups and persons with diverse interests.

THE SOVEREIGNTY OF GOD

There is yet a final factor to be included in Christian ethics: the sovereign action of the Faithful One in continuing and renewing the covenant toward righteousness and fulfillment. As the great story of Joseph, who was sold into slavery by his brothers but rose to be prime minister of Egypt and the savior of his father Jacob's family, nears its end, this passage occurs:

> After their father Jacob had died, Joseph's brothers said to one another, "What if he still has hard feelings toward us and decides now to take his revenge for the wrong we did him?" So they came to Joseph, saying, "Our father Jacob before he died said to tell you that you should forgive your brothers for their crimes against you. Now we ask your forgiveness for the crimes of the servants of the God of your father." Then his brothers wept, fell down before Joseph and declared, "We are here as your slaves." But Joseph said, "Get up. Do not be afraid. Am I to put myself in the place of God. As for you, you meant to harm me, but God intended it for good, to preserve the lives of many people. (Gen. 50:15-20)

From the faith in God that informs Christian ethics, we know that the mixtures of good and evil, individual and collective, as in the Joseph story, are not final. The Faithful One brings good even out of terrible human intentions. Assyria can become the rod of God's anger sent to punish an evil nation (Isa. 10:5-6). Habakkuk says we can perceive the historical process of purging, as one sinful nation plunders another and is in turn punished by yet another, only by climbing into a watch tower of faith. In its clearest form, the message of

God's governance is proclaimed in the tragic events of "Good" Friday. The crucifixion of Jesus Christ, exemplifying the depth of human evil, becomes in the resurrection and beyond an amazing power for liberation and fulfillment in the history of humanity. Beyond the actions of humanity, God is sovereign.

Faith and ethics in the Christian community are part of the larger story of the sovereign God, the Faithful One. We join that community and story through faith in Jesus.

NOTES

1. Mary Warnock, *Ethics Since 1900* (London: Oxford University Press, 1960), 144.
2. Ibid.
3. Johannes Althusius, The Politics of Johannes Althusius: An abridged translation of the Third Edition of POLITICA METHODICE DIGESTA, ATQUE EXEMPLIS SACRIS ET PROFANIS ILLUSTRATA. Translated, with an introduction by Frederick S. Carney (Boston: Beacon Press, 1964), 12ff.
4. The most important scholar in Christian ethics to make extensive use of other disciplines, especially the social sciences, has been H. Richard Niebuhr. For examples, see his early work, *The Social Sources of Denominationalism* (New York: Henry Holt & Co., 1929); and a late work, *The Responsible Self* (San Francisco: Harper and Row, 1963).
5. H. Richard Niebuhr, *The Meaning of Revelation* (New York: The Macmillan Company, 1941), 43.
6. See Reinhold Niebuhr, *An Interpretation of Christian Ethics* (New York: Harper and Brothers Publishers, 1935), 117ff. and passim.
7. D. Walther Eichrodt, *Theologie des alten Testaments*, Three volumes, (Leipzig: J. C. Hinrichs, 1933), vol. I, 6.
8. See Norman H. Sneath, *The Distinctive Ideas of the Old Testament* (London: Epworth Press, 1944); and Otto J. Baab, *The Theology of the Old Testament* (New York: Abingdon-Cokesbury Press, 1949).
9. Martin Buber, *The Prophetic Faith.* (New York; The Macmillan Company, 1949), passim.
10. Bernard H. Anderson, *Understanding the Old Testament* (Englewood Cliffs: Prentice-Hall, 1958), 51.
11. Simone Weil, *Waiting on God* (London: Fontana , 1959), 116.
12. James Moffatt, The Holy Bible, containing the Old and New Testaments, A New Translation (New York: Richard R. Smith, Inc., 1922).
13. Michael Polanyi, *Personal Knowledge: Towards a Post-Critical Philosophy* (Chicago: University of Chicago Press, 1958), 198-199.
14. Reinhold Niebuhr, *Moral Man and Immoral Society: A Study in Ethics and Politics* (New York: Charles Scribner's Sons, 1932), xi-xii.

15. See Charles S. McCoy and J. Wayne Baker, *Fountainhead of Federalism* (Louisville: Westminster/John Knox Press, 1991); and Carl J. Friedrich, *Trends of Federalism in Theory and Practice* (New York: Frederick A. Praeger, 1968).

16. No. 51. The quotations are taken from *The Federalist Papers*, ed. Garry Wills (New York: Bantam Books, 1982).

QUESTIONS FOR DISCUSSION

1. What do you mean when you use the word "good"?

2. What is the moral significance of *community*? To what communities do you belong?

3. What is a dichotomy? Why is the author opposed to "dichotomous thinking"?

4. How can ethics help us deal with moral ambiguity?

5. What does *commitment* or the lack of it have to do with ethics?

6. Do people typically see individualism as a problem in our contemporary society?

7. What is the importance of "story" for Christian ethics?

8. How does *covenant* play a central role in the history of Hebrew and Christian ethics? How does the author think that it should play a central role in current ethics?

9. What is the root meaning of the term "federal"? Distinguish between the meaning of the word in this essay and other meanings you may be familiar with?

10. How does the author's use of "Faithful Action" summarize his position?

PART TWO

ACROSS THE CURRICULUM

THIS IS MY JOB
FRESHMAN ENGLISH IN A POSTMODERN AGE

George Cheatham

ABSTRACT

Traditionally the study of literature has constituted cultural value or cultural capital in two senses. First, it has constituted linguistic capital, the means by which one has attained a socially credentialed and therefore valued speech. Second, it has constituted symbolic capital, a kind of knowledge-capital whose possession could be displayed upon request, thereby entitling its possessor to the cultural and material rewards of the well-educated person. The last few decades, however, have seen an undeniable decline in literature's cultural value, especially in its second sense.

Even though this decline is probably irreversible, professors of literature can respond to it in better or worse ways. I recommend an integrated curriculum of textual/historical study. Such a curriculum would, first, in broad terms, systematically question the notion that texts are somehow self-contained or self-interpreting; second, it would consequently tend to erase the long-standing disciplinary distinction between the teaching of "composition" and the teaching of "literature"; and, third, it would help students develop and acquire the skills and knowledge necessary if they are to engage in the project of emancipatory critique.

Despite its manifest humor—more likely because of it, actually—the classroom scene in the movie *National Lampoon's Animal House* (Universal 1978) generates a significant undertone of anxiety—for me, at least, and I suspect for many other teachers of college English. You may remember the scene. Professor of English literature Dave Jennings (played by Donald

Sutherland) seems helpless against the overwhelming apathy of his distracted or otherwise uninterested students. Some whisper, some doze, some doodle. The few who do seem to be trying to listen and take notes apparently have nothing to write down. He does try to engage the students and to make his text, *Paradise Lost*, seem interesting. He even uses visual aids. After asserting that Satan is the text's most interesting character, the professor writes the word *Satan* on the board, dramatically takes a bite from an apple, then asks the students if Milton was saying that being bad is more fun than being good.

But when this attempt at "relevance" fails, his pretense collapses. He in effect surrenders to the indifference. "Don't write this down," he says, then admits that Milton is long-winded and doesn't translate well into our time and confesses that he himself finds Milton as boring as Mrs. Milton found him. Of course the few earnest students do write that down; it is the one notable thing he has said. But most ignore even this confession and respond only to the bell signaling the end of class. As they are all quickly leaving without having been dismissed, he tries to talk over the noise of their departure, pleading, "But that doesn't relieve you of your responsibility for this material. I'm not kidding." Then, plaintively, his voice cracking slightly on the last word, "This is my job." Some job.

We can read this scene in a number of ways and even use it, I think, to raise a number of serious questions. The scene (actually the whole movie) generally works a sort of double move with the past. Filmed in 1978 but supposedly set in 1962, the scene both evokes and mocks a nostalgically stable and comfortable past that, the movie suggests, never really was. Most of the social and political excesses and corruptions and failures that came to be associated with the 1960s and 1970s were already present in 1962, as the film's flashforward postscript reveals. (For example, the movie's one couple will marry, we are told, then divorce five years later; the smarmy fraternity president will become an aide in the Nixon White House before being raped in prison; the overbearing ROTC officer will be killed in Vietnam by his own troops, etc.) From the perspective of literary study, the movie would have been complete had it marked Professor Jennings as a Foucauldian materialist or Derridean deconstructionist, baffling the students with talk of discursive structures, dangerous supplements, or erasure. Attending Dartmouth and Harvard in the mid-1960s, however, the movie's screenwriters (Chris Miller, Doug Kenney, Harold Ramis) would not have been exposed to such teaching.[1] As undergraduates their study of literature probably followed some version of a "Great Books" curriculum.[2]

Two points about the scene seem especially noteworthy—one, what it does not signal; the other, what it does. First, as I have just implied, the movie does not gesture toward the so-called canon war or culture war that was to erupt in the 1980s as academic postmodernism began to make its way into general public discourse. Neither Milton's dead-white-European-maleness nor *Paradise Lost*'s sexist-classist-racist-phallocentrism seems at issue. Rather the movie seems to accept indifference to Milton's epic as a given of college culture. That seems to be a large part of the joke: *Paradise Lost* is so boringly irrelevant as to be humorous on its face. Second, even so, even without any explicit gesture toward canonical or theoretical concerns, the movie manages nevertheless to mock the profession of English while clearly marking a much more serious issue than the debate over the canon. That issue is the undeniable decline since 1962 in literature's cultural status and the profession's collective anxiety over how to respond.

Even though the decline is probably irreversible, professors of literature can respond to the decline in better or worse ways. Professor Jennings' teaching represents, of course, one of the worse ways. As Mark Turner comments, "What is criminal about this scene [from *Animal House*] is that the professor has taken something that is crucially important, but not obviously so, and, by neglecting to demonstrate its importance, led the students to see the work as irrelevant and the profession as silly."[3] Turner's strong language—*criminal*—rightly suggests the ethical dimensions of the issue, which are, I think, twofold. First, as Turner suggests, is Jennings' failure adequately to represent to his students the value of Milton's text; second is his corresponding failure to use Milton's text to help his students develop the skills and acquire the knowledge necessary if they are to engage in the project of emancipatory self-reflection and, more broadly, emancipatory critique.

A better response for professors of English would be to pursue an integrated curriculum of textual/historical study—especially in freshman-level introductory courses, which, given recent enrollment trends, are the only English courses most college students will take. Such a curriculum would, first, in broad terms, systematically question the notion that texts are somehow self-contained or self-interpreting; second, it would consequently tend to erase the long-standing disciplinary division between the teaching of "composition" and the teaching of "literature"; and, third, it would, I hope, help students develop and acquire the skills and knowledge just mentioned. Before I can describe this proposed curriculum in any detail, however, I need to provide some framework. First, therefore, I will discuss the contemporary crisis in literary study, referring specifically to the ongoing canon debate and to the decline in literature's cultural value. I will then discuss John Guillory's critique of the canon debate before, finally, describing the proposed curriculum and its desired emancipatory effects.

The Crisis in Literary Study

During the last thirty or thirty-five years something has happened in this country to the study of the humanities generally and of literature specifically, something now routinely referred to as a "crisis." Certainly from our current professional perspective the study of literature thirty-five years ago seems almost quaintly untroubled and straightforward. Linguists, scholars, and critics may have had their quarrels, and competing critical methods may have been in play. But on the whole those who studied and taught literature seemed to agree on the basics of their profession. They shared certain assumptions about what they were doing and why they were doing it, shared them to such a degree that those assumptions generally remained unspoken. Such assumptions and their consequent disciplinary practices form what Thomas Kuhn has famously called a paradigm of knowledge.[4]

David Richter describes that paradigm this way:

> It was generally assumed that literary works at their best were supreme and universal expressions of the human spirit, and that students were to read these profound works in order to broaden and deepen their own humanity. The works to be studied had been sifted by time: only the greatest and most universal had survived; students reading these texts were connected with the truest and most permanent criterion of taste, the collective applause of humanity. These works were to be read closely and scrutinized carefully. It was presumed that literary meaning was more complicated than the meaning of "everyday" language, that literary texts were ambiguous or bore layers of meaning, each needing to be explored. Nevertheless, it was taken as a given that this complex of meaning was not a private meaning subjectively produced by the operations of a specific reader, but a public meaning available to any seeker.[5]

Implicit in this paradigm are the answers to three fundamental questions:

- Why do we read? To broaden and deepen our humanity, of course.
- What do we read? These infinitely valuable masterpieces, of course, known variously as Great Books, the classics, the canon.
- How do we read? With close and careful attention to the complex but publicly available meaning that is in the works themselves, of course.

The *of course* is part of any paradigm.

Robert Scholes describes the earlier paradigm similarly, but with a bit more edge, emphasizing the religious analogy implied by the word *canon*[6]:

> In our culture literature has been positioned in much the same place as scripture. We have a canon; we have exegetes who produce commentary; and, above all, we have believed that these texts contain treasures of wisdom and truth that justify the process of canonization and exegesis. When we say we "teach literature," instead of saying we teach reading, or interpretation, or criticism, we are saying that we expound the wisdom and truth of our texts, that we are in fact priests and priestesses in the service of secular scripture.[7]

So what happened to this paradigm? What, to use Scholes' words, "went wrong" with the notion of secular scripture?[8] Why don't we "teach literature" anymore?

What happened, suggests Gerald Graff, is that "theory broke out." That is to say, no longer in literary study does anything go without saying, and now anything that is spoken can be contested. To illustrate, Graff offers the following hypothetical conversation between two English professors, an Older Male Professor (OMP) and a Young Feminist Professor (YFP) concerning the ending of Matthew Arnold's poem "Dover Beach":

> Ah, love, let us be true
> To one another! For the world, which seems
> To lie before us like a land of dreams,
> So various, so beautiful, so new,
> Hath really neither joy, nor love, nor light,
> Nor certitude, nor peace, nor help for pain;
> And we are here as on a darkling plain
> Swept with confused alarms of struggle and flight
> Where ignorant armies clash by night.

Puzzled by the confusion these lines generate in his students, OMP is complaining one day in the faculty lounge. YFP, however, seems more sympathetic to the students than to OMP. In fact, she herself learned to hate poetry in high school, she says, by being forced to study "Dover Beach":

> OMP (furiously stirring his Coffee-mate): In *my* humble opinion—reactionary though I suppose it now is—"Dover Beach" is one of the great masterpieces of the Western tradition, a work that, until recently at least, every seriously educated person took for granted as part of the cultural heritage.

YFP: Perhaps, but is that altogether to the credit of the cultural heritage? Take those lines addressed to the woman. "Ah, love, let us be true to one another ..." and so forth. In other words, protect and console me, my dear—as it's the function of your naturally more spiritual sex to do—from the "struggle and flight" of politics and history that we men have been assigned the regrettable duty of dealing with.... We *should* teach "Dover Beach." But we should teach it as the example of phallocentric discourse that it is.

OMP: That's the trouble with you people; you seem to treat "Dover Beach" as if it were a piece of political propaganda rather than a work of art.... The whole point of poetry ... is to rise above such transitory issues by transmuting them into universal human experience.... "Dover Beach" is no more about gender politics than *Macbeth* is about the Stuart monarchical succession.

YFP: But *Macbeth is* about the Stuart monarchical succession, among other things—or at least its original audience may well have thought so. It's about gender politics, too: Why does Lady Macbeth have to "unsex" herself to qualify to commit murder? ... What you take to be the universal human experience in Arnold and Shakespeare ... is male experience presented as if it were universal....[9]

In this hypothetical (if exaggerated?) conversation, every significant feature of literature and the teaching of literature comes under interrogation. The questions Why read? What to read? and How to read? are all reopened, and any answer one might give is itself open to further interrogation. In Scholes' words,

> What went wrong with the idea of literature as secular scripture can be described simply as the loss of faith in the universality of human nature and a corresponding loss of faith in the universal wisdom of the authors of literary texts.[10]

The So-Called Canon War

Probably the most salient feature of the hypothetical OMP-YFP conversation is the degree to which theory, on Graff's account, points seemingly inevitably toward what has come to be called the postmodern condition, which can best be described over against Enlightenment truth-claims. According to Christopher Norris, the most important such claim is threefold:

> that human beings are able to communicate across differences of language, culture, and belief; that such communication is possible on account of their shared knowledge-constitutive interests; and moreover, that those interests have an ethical as well as a cognitive (or epistemological) bearing, since the

project of emancipatory critique is closely bound up with the capacity for distinguishing true from false—distorted or ideological—habits of belief.[11]

Postmodernism, continues Norris,

may be characterized, conversely, as a point-for-point denial of all three claims, along with an ethic (or a politics) of cultural "difference" which views Enlightenment as a discourse of unitary Truth, bent upon effacing or suppressing such heterogeneity.[12]

Of course this Enlightenment-postmodernist agon has occurred largely at an elite level among professional philosophers, social scientists, and literary critics. You can see, for example, how clearly the assertions of Graff's OMP appeal to Enlightenment claims while those of his YFP appeal to postmodernist ones. As mentioned above, however, the debate did emerge in a more general, public way as the so-called canon or culture war that broke out in the late 1980s. In this public debate ethical issues were presented, and continue to be presented, largely in the guise of ideological-political concerns. That is, the Enlightenment ethic of truth, to use Norris's words, has been argued largely in terms of traditional values and inherited ideals while the postmodernist ethic of cultural difference has been argued largely in terms of inclusivity and democratic representation. Unsurprisingly, two general factions have emerged in this public debate, roughly the political-academic right (represented, for example, by, again, Graff's OMP) and the political-academic left (represented by Graff's YFP). The basic criticism from the right is that professors no longer "teach literature," as Scholes uses the phrase above, no longer "expound the wisdom and truth of [their] texts," but instead teach politics. The basic response from the left is that all teaching is and always has been politicized—necessarily.

From the right, three books in particular have articulated the framework for a consistent and broadly appealing view. Speaking from the point of view of Graff's OMP, as it were, Allan Bloom brought canonical issues to the attention of a broad, non-specialist public with the publication of his surprise best-seller, *The Closing of the American Mind* (1987). Criticizing the contemporary liberal curriculum, Bloom argued that American colleges and universities are bringing the country into spiritual danger by their failure to teach the Great Books (Plato, Aristotle, Aquinas, Hobbes) and by their promotion instead of relativistic philosophies such as those of Weber, Nietzsche, and Dewey.[13] Roger Kimball in *Tenured Radicals* (1990) criticized not the curriculum but the contemporary liberal faculty, arguing that the student radicals of the 1960s are now the leaders of universities and are using their positions to proselytize for a leftist political agenda. Dinesh D'Souza (*Illiberal Education* 1991) argued similarly that the politicized issues of race and gender have pressured universities to admit underqualified minority students, to hire underqualified minority faculty, and to replace classic texts in the curriculum with underqualified texts, as it were, written by women and/or racial minorities.

For a seemingly arcane academic issue, this canon/culture war received extensive media coverage and at least for a while became a feature of the national political scene, especially during the general elections of 1988 and 1992. The academic issue mapped easily onto larger political-religious issues, specifically the perceived decline in so-called family values and in social and moral cohesion generally. According to traditionalists such as William Bennett, for example, politically liberal English professors, who challenged the traditional canon of great books, were at least partly responsible for the country's general moral decay and social fragmentation. Bennett in particular seemed omnipresent during the 1980s. As the director of the National Endowment for the Humanities and later Secretary of Education, he articulated a seemingly simple, no-nonsense sort of position on the canon that apparently resonated strongly with the general public.[14] Here is Bennett speaking about Western culture (and himself) in the third person:

> For some 15 to 20 years now there had been a serious degree of embarrassment, of distancing, even of repudiation of [Western] culture on the part of many of the people whose responsibility, one would think, is to transmit it. Many people in our colleges and universities aren't comfortable with the ideals of Western civilization.
>
> Bennett stands up and says, "You know, I really think people should be familiar with Homer and Shakespeare and George Eliot and Jane Austen," and they say, "We don't do that anymore. Why should we have to do that?" All right, if the purpose of the institution is not to transmit that culture, then what is the institution's purpose?[15]

Writing similarly in *Newsweek*, and perhaps sounding even more like Bennett than Bennett, political commentator George Will pushed the culture-war metaphor about as far as one can:

> The fight over [Carol] Iannone's nomination [in 1991 to the National Council on the Humanities] is particularly important precisely because you have not hitherto heard of it or her. The fight is paradigmatic of the many small skirmishes that rarely rise to public attention but cumulatively condition the nation's cultural, and then political, life. In this low-visibility, high-intensity war, [chair of the National Endowment for the Humanities] Lynne Cheney is secretary of domestic defense. The foreign adversaries her husband, Dick

[Cheney, Secretary of Defense, 1989-93], must keep at bay are less dangerous, in the long run, than the domestic forces with which she must deal. Those forces are fighting against the conservation of the common culture that is the nation's social cement. She, even more than a Supreme Court justice, deals with constitutional things. The real Constitution, which truly constitutes America, is the national mind as shaped by the intellectual legacy that gave rise to the Constitution and all the habits, mores, customs, and ideas that sustain it.[16]

The academic left has not been able to match such a media onslaught, lacking politically positioned spokespersons such as Bennett and publishing as it does generally in academic journals or in university press books rather than in, say, *Newsweek*. The general, non-specialist public has therefore not likely received a balanced view of the debate.[17] Stephen Greenblatt's response to Will's *Newsweek* article, for example, appeared in *The Chronicle of Higher Education*, a relatively specialized publication with a significantly smaller circulation. And when six leftist academics did pen a coherent response to the rightist critique, their non-best-selling manifesto (*Speaking for the Humanities* 1989) was published by the American Council of Learned Societies rather than by a mainstream publisher like Simon and Schuster, which published both Bloom and Bennett.

The basic point made in *Speaking for the Humanities*, though, is this:

The most powerful philosophies and theories have been demonstrating [that] claims of disinterestedness, objectivity, and universality are not to be trusted and themselves tend to reflect local historical conditions.[18]

On this account, objections to a politicizing of the curriculum are misguided, since any curriculum is always already politicized. Critics on the right therefore are simply objecting to politicizing the curriculum in any way but their own.

On this account, further, the Great Books curriculum has been seen as essentially conservative and hierarchically exclusive. By privileging texts written by white Anglo-Saxon males while denying status to those written by women and minorities, the traditional canon supplies a philosophical and historical foundation for a racist, sexist, and classist society. The supposed homogeneity and stability of the canon are actually the results of exclusivity and repression rather than of universality and transcendent value. In his reply to George Will, mentioned above, for example, Stephen Greenblatt, professor of Renaissance literature at Berkeley, notes the inevitable instability of artistic texts and gestures toward the necessarily active role of contemporary interpreters in the ongoing struggle over historically contested rights and values:

> [Critics such as George Will see] a wicked plot by renegade professors bent on sabotaging Western civilization by delegitimizing its founding texts and ideas. Such critics want a tame and orderly canon. The painful, messy struggles over rights and values, the political and sexual and ethical dilemmas that great art has taken upon itself to articulate and to grapple with, have no place in their curriculum. For them, what is at stake is the staunch reaffirmation of a shared and stable culture that is, as Mr. Will puts it, "the nation's social cement."
>
> But art, the art that matters, is not cement. It is mobile, complex, elusive, disturbing. A love of literature may help to forge community, but it is a community founded on imaginative freedom, the play of language, and scholarly honesty, not on flag waving, boosterism, and conformity.[19]

Perhaps the most salient feature of this public debate, though, is the degree to which it has focused (especially from the right) on the questions of Why read? and What to read? largely at the level of ideology and politics. Read classic texts, says the right, to absorb the ideals of Western civilization (an ethic of truth). Read representative texts, says the left, to recover and to acknowledge the suppressed voices of women, minorities, and other marginalized people (an ethic of cultural difference). Both kinds of texts, in other words, both classic and representative, are important in this debate largely because of what they say.

However, if we approach the question Why read? from a functionalist or materialist perspective, we get a significantly different answer, which in turn yields a significantly different answer to the question What to read? and, in addition, by foregrounding the question How to read? makes a different ethical claim. The question of whether to read a classic or a representative text is rendered secondary by a curriculum of textual/historical study. Primary in such a curriculum is the focus on reading in such a way as to foster emancipatory critique (an ethic of critique) as a third, middle approach. Before discussing these points in more detail, however, I must first discuss the decline of literature.

The Decline of Literature

To return for a moment to the classroom scene from *Animal House*, the fact that Professor Jennings is teaching a canonical text seems irrelevant. Instead of *Paradise Lost* he could be teaching Frederick Douglass's *Narrative of the Life* or *I Rigoberta Menchu* (the autobiography of a female Guatemalan revolutionary included on the infamous revised Western Civilization reading list at Stanford).[20] It would not much matter. What seems more significant than what is being read is, first, the classroom setting itself, the institutionalized site of reading, and, second, as I said earlier, the evident decline in literature's cultural status since the movie's setting in 1962.

For one thing, a smaller percentage of college students even sit in literature classrooms now than did in the mid-1960s. Richard Ohmann, for example, notes this obvious falling off:

> Majors in English and allied fields are down 50 percent or more in two decades [prior to 1990]. Departments have shrunk. Recent estimates suggest that from 15 to 40 percent of job seekers in our field find permanent employment there. And the students still in our classrooms are mostly studying composition, which accounted for 40 percent of English enrollments in the late 1960s; it accounts for 60 percent now, and for twice the number of literature enrollments.[21]

Why? Mostly, says Ohmann, because students perceive that degrees in English and allied fields will not much help them get jobs:

> I see no evidence that students derive less benefit from the study of literature, or are less attracted to that study, now than in 1965. Rather, it seems to me that the statistics tell a simple story: students will pursue an inherently pleasant and humane activity when there is no penalty for doing so, as in the 1960s when there was a shortage of educated workers and every BA got a job.... These circumstances underscore the folly of discussing our profession in an historical vacuum. The market determines the use of our work by a calculus of exchange value that need not correspond to our own use values, and right now we—or I should say, our students and younger colleagues—are experiencing one of the irrationalities, a minor but painful one, of the market system.[22]

In his critique of the canon debate, *Cultural Capital: The Problem of Literary Canon Formation* (1993), John Guillory explores at length this notion of literature's market value that Ohmann refers to. He argues persuasively that the decline in the percentage of students studying literature reflects a decline in the value of literary currency, as it were. In fact, the canon debate, says Guillory, "signifies nothing less than a crisis in the form of cultural capital we call 'literature.'"[23] (One great irony of the canon debate is the fact that the sorts of curricular revisions deplored by conservatives such as Bennett and Will seem to be, on Guillory's account, driven more by free market capitalism than by leftist political ideology.) And the decline in enrollments exemplifies what Guillory calls "cultural capital flight":

> The professional-managerial class has made the correct assessment that, so far as its future profit is concerned, the reading of great works is not worth the investment of very much time or money. The perceived devaluation of the humanities curriculum is in reality a decline in its *market* value. If the liberal arts curriculum still survives as the preferred course of study in some elite institutions, this fact has everything to do with the class constituency of these institutions. With few exceptions, it is only those students who belong to the financially secure upper classes who do not feel compelled to acquire professional or technical knowledge as undergraduates. The professional-managerial class, on the other hand, many of whose members have only recently attained to middle and upper-middle class status, depends entirely on the acquisition of technical knowledge in order to maintain its status, or to become upwardly mobile.[24]

The term cultural capital is a class-based concept that Guillory takes from the work of neo-Marxist sociologist Pierre Bourdieu and applies to the problem of canon formation. In the case of the literary curriculum, says Guillory, "the problem of what is called canon formation is best understood as a problem in the constitution and distribution of cultural capital, or more specifically, a problem of access to the means of literary production and consumption."[25] On this account, the particular works read are of significantly less importance than is the institutional site at which they are read, the school, "which regulates access to literary production by regulating access to literacy, to the practices of reading and writing."[26]

Thus, continues Guillory:

> The literary syllabus is the institutional form by means of which this knowledge [literacy] is disseminated, and it constitutes capital in two senses: First, it is *linguistic* capital, the means by which one attains to a socially credentialed and therefore valued speech, otherwise known as "Standard English." And second, it is *symbolic* capital, a kind of knowledge-capital whose possession can be displayed upon request and which thereby entitles its possessor to the cultural and material rewards of the well-educated person.[27]

It is this value of both literature's linguistic and symbolic capital that has declined. As Guillory bluntly puts it, the cultural capital of literature is becoming "increasingly marginal to the social function of the present educational system."[28] The students in *Animal House* seem to know, or at least intuit, that the reading of literature is not worth the investment of much effort. Hence their apathy. And hence, too, the discrepancy between the number of students enrolled in literature classes and in composition classes. As the professional-managerial class knows, literature is no longer the means to attain a "socially credentialed and therefore valued speech." This change is one reason for the crisis in the literary syllabus; that syllabus can no longer be seen as speaking and disseminating a language that aspires to "universality." That educational task has been assumed, instead, by the syllabus of composition. Says Guillory, "The students who regard composition as a necessary prerequisite for entry into professional life know this, without knowing what it is that they know."[29]

GUILLORY'S CRITIQUE OF THE CANON DEBATE

On Guillory's account, then, the debate over whether to teach "canonical" or "non-canonical" literature has both 1) masked the long-term decline in the cultural capital of literature (which gave rise to the debate in the first place) and 2) all along been a sort of false debate. That is, the distinction between canonical and non-canonical literature has developed through a process involving the de-historicizing of literary categories and a misreading of the effect of the syllabus as an institutional instrument. To illustrate this latter point, we might look briefly at a section of the pre-revision reading list for Stanford's course in Western Civilization, the section titled the "Ancient World":[30]

Required:	Strongly Recommended:
Hebrew Bible, Genesis	Thucydides
Plato, *Republic*, major portions of books 1-7	Aristotle, *Nicomachean Ethics*, *Politics*
Homer, major selections from *Iliad*, *Odyssey*, or both	Cicero
At least one Greek tragedy	Virgil, *Aeneid*
New Testament, selections including a gospel	Tacitus

How does such a list relate to the canon? Ovid is not on this list. Nor are two of the three major Greek tragedians. Nor are most of the Hebrew Bible and New Testament. Are these omitted texts, then, non-canonical? Or, not being included on the list, do they have any status at all?

Such questions do not really take us very far, Guillory suggests, for they make two basic mistakes. First, they allow for only two categories of literary works (canonical/non-canonical) when the historical context makes clear that literature is actually "a complex continuum of major works, minor works, works read primarily in research contexts, works as yet simply shelved in the archive."[31] The degree to which we conventionally recognize as canonical only those works taught in literature survey courses or included in anthologies, however, suggests the degree to which the debate about the canon has been de-historicized and has been driven by institutional agendas.[32]

Second, such questions confuse "the syllabus, a selection of texts for study in a particular institutional context, with the canon itself—the sum total of works supposed to be 'great.'"[33] Since any syllabus is necessarily limited by the constraints of a particular college course and its rubric, the "canon" itself is never the object of study in any classroom. But if that is the case, where, then, does the canon appear? Nowhere, exactly, says Guillory, for

> the canon is an *imaginary* totality of works. No one has access to the canon as a totality. This fact is true in the trivial sense that no one ever reads every canonical work; no one can, because the works invoked as canonical change continually according to many different occasions of judgment or contestation. What this means is that the canon is never other than an imaginary list; it never appears as a complete and uncontested list in any particular time and place, not even in the form of the omnibus anthology, which remains a selection from a larger list.... . In this context, the distinction between the canonical and the non-canonical can be seen not as the form in which judgments are actually made about individual works, but as an effect of the syllabus as an institutional instrument... . [T]he syllabus posits the existence of the canon as its imaginary totality. The imaginary list is projected out of the multiple individual syllabi functioning within individual pedagogic institutions over a relatively extended period of time. Changing the syllabus cannot mean in any historical context overthrowing the canon, because every construction of a syllabus *institutes* once again the process of canon formation.[34]

These two mistakes tend, as well, to have a flattening or homogenizing effect on texts. That is, the institutionalized syllabus/canon both generates a specious unity by suggesting a whole from which representative texts have been selected and retroactively constructs its individual texts as a tradition. If unchecked the end product of such institutionalization is the fetishized list of "Great Books" or "Ideals of Western Civilization." "If a principle of specious unity is implicit in the construction of any syllabus," says Guillory,

> this means that the form of the syllabus sets up the conditions within which it is possible to forget that the syllabus is just a list, that there is no concrete cultural totality of which it is the expression. The confusion of the syllabus with the canon thus inaugurates a pedagogy of misreading, wherein a given text's historical specificity is effaced as it is absorbed into the unity of the syllabus/canon.[35]

The way to avoid such absorption, continues Guillory, is to teach not the kinds of information that can be transmitted by a list but the kinds of knowledge and skills (detailed below) that will enable students to make sense of a list, that will enable them to understand the systemic relations among the items on the list that have constructed the list as constitutive of that cultural capital that we call, for example, Great Books in the first place.

Proposed Curriculum of Textual/Historical Study

If Guillory is correct—and I believe he is—then why and how we teach literature are of far greater consequence than what we teach. But why and how should we teach whatever texts it is that we do choose? The introductory English and history courses already required at most liberal arts colleges could relatively easily be reconfigured into a coordinated freshman-year curriculum of textual/historical study that would answer both of these questions.[36] Understandably, since I am a professor of English, my emphasis here will be on the English rather than the history courses. In constructing these proposed courses, I draw on Guillory's critique of the canon in *Cultural Capital*, Robert Scholes' critique of what he calls "the English apparatus" in *Textual Power: Literary Theory and the Teaching of English*, and Cornel West's call for democratic pragmatism in "Pragmatism and the Tragic." More specifically, from Guillory I take the notion of historicity; from Scholes I take the notion of textuality; and from West I take an overarching structure.

How to Teach the Required English Courses

The reconfigured English courses, along with the history, would, ideally, embody what Guillory calls "an integrated curriculum of textual/historical study"[37] and what Scholes calls "textuality."[38] Such courses would attempt to bridge the literature/composition gap by emphasizing textual knowledge and textual skills rather than emphasizing self-contained works (as the Great Books approach invites). The texts studied in these courses need not be literature in the traditional sense (although they could, and some will, be), nor need they be canonical in the traditional sense (although they could, and some will, be). But they should be studied intertextually. That is, they should be studied not as self-contained or self-interpreting works but as texts necessarily enmeshed in a network of relations with other texts and institutional practices. As Scholes puts it, the point is "to make the object of study the whole intertextual system of relations that connects one text to others—a system that will finally include the student's own writing."[39]

Reading, on this account, is what Scholes calls a "textual economy, in which pleasure and power are exchanged between producers and consumers of texts, always remembering that writers must consume in order to produce and that readers must produce in order to consume."[40] In giving us pleasure texts exercise power over us, and the experience of textual pleasure always entails some loss of sovereignty on the readers' part, some surrender to the text. An understanding of how texts work, however, an understanding of the discursive and rhetorical structures that enable texts both to generate pleasure and to exert power allows us to resist texts through our own analytic labor and to exert our own power against them by creating our own critical texts, a process that generates a pleasure of its own. In such a complex dynamic of power and pleasure, students both find and to some extent construct their selves through encountering a textualized other, whose existence must be respected. The reading self, willing to question its own certitude, dialectically encounters a textualized other beset, like the reader her- or himself, by the complexities of human existence.

A curriculum of textual/historical study would thus necessarily contextualize texts, uncovering their historical and cultural specificity and foregrounding the mechanisms by which meaning and value are discursively constructed. The proposed courses, therefore, would not be masterpiece-driven survey courses or anthology-driven introductions to literature. Even though the masterpiece/anthology approach is good at providing "coverage," it tends to foreground the "workness" of texts and to mask their intertextuality. Remember, for example, William Bennett's call to "transmit" Western Culture by making students "familiar with" Homer, etc., as if Western Culture were somehow simply there in the *Iliad* and somehow directly accessible through an uncertainly defined familiarity. The notion that culture can be transparently contained in and transparently transmitted through texts is what textual/historical study above all seeks to critique.

To foreground instead the intertextual system of relations, Scholes suggests introducing students to the study of literature not with anthologies of masterpieces but with collections of works by the same author—a collection of short stories by Joyce, for example, rather than an anthology of short stories by different authors. These English courses would not be, however, simply introductions to the study of literature. Therefore I suggest a different configuration of texts than Scholes.

WHAT TEXTS TO STUDY
IN THE REQUIRED ENGLISH COURSES

The proposed English courses would work better if organized according to some overarching structure or theme that could map easily onto the syllabus of American history. One such theme is suggested by Cornel West, who argues that the tradition of American pragmatism "has to do with trying to conceive of knowledge, reality and truth in such a way that it promotes the flowering and flourishing of individuality under conditions of democracy."[41] This tradition, he continues, has shaped American history and has "laid the foundation for the meaning and value of democracy in America in the modern world."[42] West names as the "grand spiritual godfathers of pragmatism" Jefferson, Emerson, and Lincoln.[43] I do not think that students in freshman English should necessarily study something so specific as the tradition of American pragmatism (although they could). However, West's emphasis on the conditions of democracy (which echoes Guillory), along with his naming of three seminal figures, suggests a theme and a structure and thus organizational criteria for the selection of texts.

First, the texts selected for study would map onto the background and chronology of American history. Not inconsequentially, such a structure should be evident to students and thus should provide a sort of scaffolding for them. Such a structure should further suggest to students a reason for the study of an individual text and should render more accessible the historical specificity of that individual text. In addition, a truly integrated curriculum of textual/historical study would link the required English courses directly to freshman-level courses in American history, such that every student enrolled in first- or second-semester English would be concurrently enrolled in first- or second-semester American history.

Second, as mentioned above, the texts studied would not be Great Books-like or anthology-like texts. Instead they would be what I will call clustered texts. By that I mean that they might be multiple contemporary texts responding to the same historical or social conditions or they might be texts engaged in conversation with each other. Those texts would cluster, moreover, around significant or nodal issues in American history. Although it does not greatly matter which specific issues are chosen or which specific texts, those that have played the largest parts in our ongoing national conversation are obvious choices. The primary criterion is that the issues and texts foreground the project of emancipatory critique.

For example, I would have students read the Declaration of Independence—a canonical, seminal, even sacred American text—but I would not have them read it in isolation. Instead they would read it along with some of the ninety-odd other, local declarations of independence that preceded the "real" one. These other declarations are detailed in Pauline Maier's recent book, *American Scripture: Making the Declaration of Independence*, where she uses them to question, among other things, the role of individual genius in the composition of the national document. She emphasizes the group revision performed on Jefferson's draft, for instance, and notes the degree to which Jefferson's language echoes that of the many local declarations. Jefferson was especially influenced, says Maier, by George Mason's "Declaration of Rights," drafted to serve as part of Virginia's declaration of state independence and published in a Philadelphia newspaper where Jefferson read it. Mason wrote "that all men are born equally free and independent, and have certain inherent natural rights, of which they cannot, by any compact, deprive or divest their posterity; among which are the enjoyment of life and liberty, with the means of acquiring and possessing property, and pursuing and obtaining happiness and safety."[44] Maier also traces the process by which the Declaration eventually came to be regarded as American scripture—specifically the history of attitudes toward the document and toward its authorship. In short, Maier does to the Declaration just those sorts of things that an integrated curriculum of textual/historical study should do.

Thus, to mimic Maier, I would have the students read—and write in response to—one or two of the local declarations, Mason's declaration, Jefferson's draft declaration, the final revised declaration, perhaps an excerpt from Maier's book, and perhaps something like Frederick Douglass's essay "What to the Slave Is the Fourth of July?" This reading and writing about the Declaration of Independence, of course, would complement the reading and writing being done in the students' concurrent course in American history. The point is that the students would read the Declaration of Independence not as a transcendently self-contained and self-interpreting work—and not even as a work with a historical background—but as a text enmeshed with other texts (including their own) and with institutional and historical practices.

Third, ideally, as suggested by West and by my discussion of Maier, the texts studied would cohere in such a way as *both* to interrogate *and* to promote the flowering and flourishing of individualism under conditions of democracy. Paradigmatic in this respect would be Douglass's "What to the Slave Is the Fourth of July?"

WHY TEACH THE REQUIRED ENGLISH COURSES THIS WAY

Why should we teach freshman-year English as an integrated curriculum of textual/historical study? The short answer is, to set our students free—free to read and rewrite inherited texts within the contexts of their own lives. As Scholes elaborates,

> The students who come to us now exist in the most manipulative culture human beings have ever experienced. They are bombarded with signs, with rhetoric, from their daily awakenings until their troubled sleep, especially with signs transmitted by the audio-visual media. And, for a variety of reasons, they are relatively deprived of experience in the thoughtful reading and writing of verbal texts. They are also sadly deficient in certain kinds of historical knowledge that might give them some perspective on the manipulation they currently encounter.
> What students need from us ... now is the kind of knowledge and skill that will enable them to make sense of their worlds, to determine their own interests, both individual and collective, to see through the manipulations of all sorts of texts in all sorts of media, and to express their own views in some appropriate manner.[45]

Guillory offers a similar rationale. A "necessary social condition of democracy," he says, "is the general exercise of a certain kind of intellectual labor, and ... a specific body of knowledge ... is the necessary medium in the schools for the exercise of this intellectual labor."[46] That body of knowledge, he says, is not the specific kinds of "information" or "culture" specified, for example, by E.D. Hirsch in his best-selling *Dictionary of Cultural Literacy*. Instead it is the study of cultural texts (described above) as a practice of reading and writing. And by intellectual labor he means the sort of critical thinking enabled by such knowledge. Such knowledge, says Guillory, will not guarantee critical thinking or democracy, but such knowledge is a necessary condition for their realization.

Earlier I quoted Christopher Norris's definition of postmodernism in contradistinction to Enlightenment, a definition that, as Norris knows, both simplifies and overstates their differences. Unfortunately, as is evident from the preceding discussion, such simplification and overstatement pervade the debate over what to teach in college-level English courses, especially in its non-specialist, public version. But we do not have to settle for either Truth with a capital *T* or, lacking such Truth, a reflexive slide toward a wholesale negative ontology. Yes, the Enlightenment paradigm in its extreme form does imply a privileged and suppressive Truth, and, yes, the corrosive skepticism of extreme postmodernism does threaten to flatten into impotence and indifference. But extremes can, I think, meet. After all, one of the Enlightenment's principal achievements is the protocols it developed for the questioning of received ideas and values, including its own. And even Jacques Derrida, perhaps the chief proponent of postmodernism, has argued all along that one cannot escape traditional Enlightenment concepts such as truth and rigor but instead can only use such concepts to interrogate the tradition's blind spots.

Such knowledge and intellectual labor as described above by Scholes and Guillory—and practiced by Derrida, among many others—constitute the ongoing project of emancipatory self-reflection and critique. A knowledge of inherited canons and protocols, along with an understanding of how such canons and protocols have been historically and discursively constructed, gives us the freedom to question received ideas and values and to continue to seek the truth based on the best canons and protocols we can continue to construct. Our ethical challenge as professors of English is to stake out a position—and through a curriculum of textual/historical study to equip our students to stake out a position—in this difficult middle terrain.

Coda

"Fat, drunk, and stupid is no way to go through life, son." At least this is what Dean Wormer explains to Flounder, a freshman at *Animal House*'s Faber College who is flunking out after only one semester. What, I wonder, could Professor Jennings have done to help this pitiful student? (During Jennings' class Flounder is shown excitedly drawing jet aircraft strafing enemy soldiers.) I suppose the obesity and inebriation are beyond Jennings' professional reach. But the stupidity? Who knows? Had Faber offered an integrated curriculum of textual/historical study, the professor—and the student—might at least have had a fighting chance. But that would not have made a very funny movie.

NOTES

1. Yale and Johns Hopkins Universities generally spearheaded the introduction of continental-style literary theory into the American English curriculum during the early to mid-1970s. Dartmouth and Harvard were relatively slow to adopt.
2. As I explain later in the text, the term Great Books generally suggests a collection of literary masterpieces thought to express universal truths of the human condition.
3. Mark Turner, *Reading Minds: The Study of English in the Age of Cognitive Science* (Princeton: Princeton University Press, 1991), 5. Although Turner first brought my attention to this scene from the movie, I read the scene differently than he does.
4. Thomas Kuhn, *The Structure of Scientific Revolutions*, 2nd ed. (Chicago: University of Chicago Press, 1970), 10.
5. David Richter, *Falling into Theory: Conflicting Views on Reading Literature* (Boston: St. Martin's, 1994), 2. This whole section of my paper owes much to Richter.
6. The word *canon* derives from two Greek words: *kanna* meaning reed and *kanon* meaning a measuring line or rule. It entered English usage through the Latin of the Catholic Church, where *canon* came primarily to name the body of church law and to designate the books of scripture officially accepted as genuine. Only recently in literary study has the term generally replaced *classics* as a designation for the totality of literary texts recognized as great.
7. Robert Scholes, *Textual Power: Literary Theory and the Teaching of English* (New Haven: Yale University Press, 1985), 12-13.
8. Ibid., 13.
9. Gerald Graff, *Professing Literature: An Institutional History* (Chicago: University of Chicago Press, 1987), 38-39.
10. Scholes, *Textual Power*, 13.
11. Christopher Norris, *Truth and the Ethics of Criticism* (Manchester: Manchester University Press, 1994), 32.
12. Ibid.
13. It is perhaps worth noting that Bloom's book focuses largely on philosophical rather than literary texts.
14. Indeed, Bennett has developed his traditionalist position into a veritable cottage industry of morality, issuing four best-selling collections of moral tales: *The Book of Virtues: A Treasury of Great Moral Stories* (New York: Simon and Schuster, 1988); *The Children's Book of Virtues* (New York: Simon and Schuster, 1995); *The Moral Compass: Stories for a Life's Journey* (New York: Simon and Schuster, 1995); and *Our Sacred Honor: Words of Advice from the Founders in Stories, Letters, Poems, and Speeches* (New York: Simon and Schuster, 1997).
15. William Bennett, Editorial, *New York Times*, 17 February 1985, quoted in John Guillory, *Cultural Capital* (Chicago: University of Chicago Press, 1993), 20.
16. George Will, "Literary Politics," in *Falling into Theory*, ed. David Richter (Boston: St. Martin's, 1994), 288.
17. In *Cultural Selection* (New York: Basic Books, 1997) Gary Taylor suggests that popular support in such matters will always be with the traditionalists rather than the revisionists, who are always specialists:

> The growing discrepancy between artificial and biological memory has created an increasing conflict between tradition and the editorial specialists who investigate artificial memories of the past [such as literary texts]. More and more often, more and more insistently, individuals in our culture are called upon to alter their memories of the past, as the traumatic memories our culture had chosen to forget have been recollected. We are inundated by the return of memories we had repressed.... The most important ideological conflicts of the last five centuries—including the "culture wars" of the last fifteen years—have been driven by emotional resistance to the artificial recovery of repressed memories. (219-20)

Taylor goes on to catalog twelve "simple reactions" that characterize the traditionalists' defense mechanisms (220-35). A useful exercise is to read William Bennett and George Will, for example, against this catalog.

18. George Levine, et al., *Speaking for the Humanities* (New York: American Council of Learned Societies, 1989), 18.

19. Stephen Greenblatt, "The Politics of Culture," in *Falling into Theory*, ed. David Richter (Boston: St. Martin's, 1994), 289-90.

20. In 1988 the faculty of Stanford University debated a proposed revision of its Western Civilization course. The debate attracted the attention of professional traditionalists such as William Bennett, George Will, and William F. Buckley. See Mary Louise Pratt, for example, "Humanities for the Future: Reflections on the Western Culture Debate at Stanford," *South Atlantic Quarterly* 89 (1990): 7-25. Stanford first offered a Western Civilization course in 1935 but abolished the requirement about 1970. In 1978 the university began a two-year pilot program to reinstitute the course, and in 1980 it required the year-long course of all incoming freshmen. The course was structured around a reading list (see below) that emphasized self-contained works and reflected what Pratt calls a Eurocentric narrative of origins. (That is, from its birth in classical Greece and Rome, Western civilization moved through the Italian renaissance and the Franco-German enlightenment on its way to becoming European lettered high culture.) The Stanford faculty voted to continue offering the course but to allow also for other tracks structured around other understandings of culture or broader perspectives of the West. One alternative track, for example, called Europe and the Americas, incorporated European, African, and native American strands of American cultures and the history of their interactions in the Americas. One of the texts read in this alternative track was *I Rigoberta Menchu*.

Section one of the pre-revised reading list (the Ancient World) is reproduced in my text. Here are the other two sections:

Medieval and Renaissance

Required:
- Augustine, *Confessions*, 1-9
- Dante, *Inferno*
- More, *Utopia*
- Machiavelli, *The Prince*
- Luther, *Christian Liberty*
- Galileo, *The Starry Messenger, The Assayer*

Strongly recommended:
- Boethius, *Consolation of Philosophy*
- Aquinas, selections
- A Shakespearean tragedy
- Cervantes, *Don Quixote*
- Descartes, *Discourse on Method, Meditations*
- Hobbes, *Leviathan*
- Locke, *Second Treatise of Civil Government*

	Modern
Required:	Strongly recommended:
Voltaire, *Candide*	Rousseau, *Social Contract,*
Marx and Engels, *Communist Manifesto*	*Confessions, Emile*
	Hume, *Enquiries, Dialogues on Natural Religion*
Freud, *Outline of Psychoanalysis, Civilization and Its Discontents*	Goethe, *Faust, Sorrows of Young Werther*
Darwin, selections	Nineteenth-century novel
	Mill, *Essay on Liberty, The Subjection of Women*
	Nietzsche, *Genealogy of Morals, Beyond Good and Evil*

21. Richard Ohmann, "The Function of English at the Present Time," in *Falling into Theory*, ed. David Richter (Boston: St. Martin's, 1994), 100-05.
22. Ibid., 103.
23. John Guillory, *Cultural Capital: The Problem of Literary Canon Formation* (Chicago: University of Chicago Press, 1993), *viii*.
24. Ibid., 46.
25. Ibid., *ix*.
26. Ibid.
27. Ibid.
28. Ibid., *x*.
29. Ibid., 81.
30. Ibid., 31.
31. Ibid., 30.
32. In the classroom, as an obvious example, a one-volume anthology of masterpieces is both more economical and more convenient than other kinds of textbooks. Thus the material facts of institutionalized book publishing tend to support the notion of the self-contained masterpiece. This support is compounded, moreover, by the ease with which a collection of self-contained masterpieces maps logically onto the syllabus of a sixteen-week semester divided into relatively self-contained fifty-minute class periods.
33. Guillory, 29.
34. Ibid., 30-31.
35. Ibid., 34.
36. My own school, for example, Greensboro College, requires two English courses of all students during the freshman year: ENG 101, Academic Discourse I, and ENG 102, Academic Discourse/Literature II. And it requires two history courses of all students chosen from these four: HIST 141, History of the United States I; HIST 142, History of the United States II; HIST 101, World History I; and HIST 102, World History II. Without much curricular disruption and without adding to the overall number of general education requirements, the College could require four coordinated freshman-year courses of English and American history.
37. Guillory, 54.
38. Scholes, *Textual Power*, 20.
39. Ibid., 31.

40. Robert Scholes, *Protocols of Reading* (New Haven: Yale University Press, 1989), 90.
41. Cornel West, *Prophetic Thought in Postmodern Times* (Monroe, ME: Common Courage Press, 1993), 32.
42. Ibid.
43. Ibid.
44. Pauline Maier, *American Scripture: Making the Declaration of Independence* (New York: Knopf, 1997), quoted in Alan Taylor, "Pluribus," *The New Republic*, 30 June 1997, 35.
45. Scholes, *Textual Power*, 15-16.
46. Guillory, 51.

QUESTIONS FOR DISCUSSION

1. Is the decline in literature's cultural status only linked to its lack of "market value"? What role does an anti-intellectual culture play in such a decline?

2. If how and why we teach became as important or more important than what we teach, do professors have an obligation to share their reasoning, decision making, problem solving, and thinking processes with their students?

3. What impact does the shift from *what* is taught to *how* and *why* we teach, have upon the expertise, authority, and power relationships between professors and students?

4. How would professors supporting a historical/textual study share their goals with their students? Specifically, how will students determine their own interests and make sense of their world? In an integrated curriculum of textual/historical study, should students be included in the syllabus constructing process?

5. Can a particular curriculum, course of study, or pedagogy generate desired character attributes such as intellectual curiosity, critical consciousness, or individual creativity?

6. What interests of the political right are being maintained by the canon? What interests of the left are upheld by the integrated, textual/historical curriculum? How does a sense of what is integral to Western civilization play a part in this cultural-curricular-canonical debate?

9. What is a classic? Who or what makes this determination?

THE VALUE OF LITERATURE IN AN ETHICS ACROSS THE CURRICULUM PROGRAM OF A LIBERAL ARTS COLLEGE

Charles Hebert

ABSTRACT

While the English teaching area must recognize that it cannot be all things to all people, a focused emphasis on the texts of major authors could enhance students' ability to think critically and act ethically. A course content change in the required English classes at liberal arts colleges could greatly enhance an English teaching area's contribution to the study of ethics. Having students read texts of major authors would help these students understand themselves so they might act thoughtfully and thus be better prepared to live as more humane, responsible, and productive members of society.

Having students read literature from major authors not only helps these students learn to think critically but also to gain insights into the human condition. Over the last three decades, the trend in first-year English classes has been to move away from the use of literature, with the emphasis shifted to rhetoric and composition. What that does, it seems to me, is to remove the ethical dimensions presented through the great works.

THE PROBLEM

The content of most introductory English classes, even more than that of other "service" courses at liberal arts colleges, is usually determined as much by the needs of the academic community as by the desires of the faculty teaching those classes. These introductory English courses primarily certify that first-year students possess at least the minimum communication skills necessary for success with college-level work: to read and view intelligently, to write and speak articulately, and, perhaps, most importantly, to think critically. And, as if these responsibilities were not already enough, the advent of technology and the subsequent need for computer literacy in all of its manifestations have begun to put increasing pressure on the content of the introductory English courses. Admittedly, students who do not arrive at college with a knowledge of electronic communication skills must learn them somewhere. And, yes, electronic communication is communication, requiring articulation in language. Therefore, who better to assure that first-year students have the basics so essential for success at college than those people with the purported expertise in language?

But an English teaching area at a liberal arts college cannot be all things to all people. Students are not being served well if the content of English classes becomes so diverse that we neglect the responsibility to teach students to think critically about the information they receive, and then to articulate the result of their analyses. But if there is already a problem with the complex variety of diverse ingredients that constitute introductory English classes, any attempt to blend yet another ingredient, ethics, into this already overloaded mix would seem sheer insanity.

THE SOLUTION

However, a change in the focus of introductory English classes to emphasize once again the study of literature could possibly effect a beneficial solution. As John Guillory explains, the social function of the schools has long been, among other things, to produce a distinction between a basic and a more elite language; the ongoing shift from "literature" to "composition" reflects a shift in how we as a culture define basic and elite language. As Guillory uses the term, literary language—characterized by its reflection of the style, grammar and syntax, and range of reference—also deals with the ideological concerns of canonical literature (Chaucer, Shakespeare, Dante, Milton,

Wordsworth, Tennyson, Melville, Whitman, James, for example). By the language of composition, on the other hand, Guillory means the standard vernacular English of the professional-managerial classes.[1] Whether the current pressure on the college curriculum reflects the schools' failure to teach standard vernacular English (and electronic communication skills) at the lower levels of the educational system or whether some other factor explains this shift in emphasis is moot.[2] Whatever the causes, the trend has the unfortunate effect of pushing the study of literature out of introductory English classes. As composition theorist Edward Corbet has bluntly stated, "[L]iterary texts will more often than not serve as a distraction from rather than a promoter of the objectives of a writing course."[3]

THE CONSEQUENCES

The effect of this trend to devalue literature is especially unfortunate for liberal arts colleges. What good literature can do and has done well in the past is (1) to educate people to think critically so that they can better understand, evaluate, and apply information and (2) to present "life" with all its dimensions and moral dilemmas so that people are able to learn to improve themselves through the "experiences" of others. As John Gardner maintains in *On Moral Fiction*, "True art [which includes literature] is moral: it seeks to improve life, not to debase it. It seeks to hold off, at least for a while, the twilight of the gods and us."[4]

If students are not trained to understand properly the information presented to them so that they can formulate their own value judgments, then they will be at the mercy of whoever controls the information. They cannot be expected to be able to form adequate value judgments until they have an adequate understanding of what is commonly referred to as "the human condition." Too many people are willing to leave ethics to the study of philosophy and religion when in actuality great literature presents a world of possibilities for explorations in ethics. As Adeimantus says to Socrates in Plato's *Republic*:

> [T]hose who take up philosophy—not those who merely dabble in it while still young in order to complete their upbringing and then drop it, but those who continue in it for a longer time—the greatest number become cranks, not to say completely vicious, while those who seem completely decent are rendered useless.... (487d)

Socrates agrees with this assessment, claiming the philosopher has not been raised under the right sort of constitution: "Under a suitable one, his own growth would be fuller, and he'll save the community as well as himself" (497a). Most of us are still waiting. Our present rulers do not possess the wisdom of Plato's guardians, but neither do the fields of religion and philosophy have exclusive domain. All citizens have an obligation to learn how to make good moral choices. To paraphrase a popular quip, ethics is much too important to be left in the hands of the experts. That, of course, is one of the goals of Ethics Across the Curriculum in a liberal arts setting.

But there is an additional problem. As David Denby, who recently returned to Columbia University to repeat two courses in the Western classics that he had first taken as a freshman in 1961, observes, "[T]here is only one 'hegemonic discourse' in the lives of American undergraduates, and that is the mass media. Most [educators] can't begin to compete against the torrent of imagery and sound that makes every moment but the present seem quaint, bloodless, or dead."[5] Literature cannot hope to best the incessant hype of the mass media. Trying to find easier and more "user-friendly" readings for students accomplishes only a further degeneration of learning. Instead, we need to counter the "hegemonic discourse" of the mass media by exposing students to texts that correspond to Harold Bloom's definition of the canonical: "One ancient test for the canonical remains fiercely valid: unless it demands rereading, the work does not qualify... . Contra certain Parisians, the text is there to give not pleasure but the high unpleasure or more difficult pleasure that a lesser text will not provide."[6] "User-friendly" readings that students can digest without effort will do little to counter the onslaught of the mass media's intellectual assault, especially the vast array of immediate, although often unreliable, information on the Internet.

However, the discipline that comes from confronting a difficult text from another kind of culture (and most past texts are) is invaluable in countering the pervasive allure of the mass media and the siren call of technology for the sake of innovation.[7] Although Plato banished "false poetry" from his perfect republic, we cannot and should not restrict student access to information. The ethical thing, however, is to introduce students to those great writers of the past who deal with the difficult issues that beset the human condition. In addition, students should be provided the opportunity to become familiar with at least some of the major writers and, in the process, also be taught the critical thinking skills necessary to make valid judgments about information. Information presented to people without critical thinking skills is as likely to produce Nazis or Heaven's Gate cultists as it is to produce good citizens, if one is so inclined. A change in the approach to introductory English classes that would reflect ethical issues could be part of the solution instead of an addition to the problem; part of what is missing from what students need stems from the content of the introductory courses themselves.

THE MISSING PIECE

First-year English programs need to embrace literature once more. Literature, the missing piece, has been long believed to be an effective weapon in this all-important struggle "against the twilight"[8] to which Gardner refers. No permanent master list of "Great Books" need be formulated. The faculty members on a particular campus merely need to identify authors who share the ethical values exemplified in their mission statement. As Dennis O'Brien, the president emeritus of the University of Rochester, observes in "The Disappearing Moral Curriculum":

> In our contemporary culture wars, the lesson from the 19th-century college is that a canon is indispensable if one is to develop a critical and rational eye for morality. Education from a canon of classics is open-textured, admitting new "classics" and different "traditions," but a canon cannot be wholly abandoned. "Canonic" studies become problematic when the canon gets frozen around *the* exemplary... or when a canon is consigned to some cultic cave (the multiculturalist temptation). It is quite legitimate to argue about what should be in the canon, for there are always marginal works, and former classics may be outclassed by historical development, but in morality, as in music, setting the canon may be the most serious task of the educator.[9]

Simply working to establish better communication among the faculty to determine what authors the faculty as a whole, not just the English faculty, deem important to a liberally educated graduate could easily facilitate creating a diverse and variable body of literature.

Considerable thought should be given as faculty formulate their own list of authors from those in the current intellectual conversation who would be useful to students. Some faculty might determine appropriate authors from those cited by journalists, political leaders, and public policy makers. Others may turn to the more traditional authors: Plato, Socrates, Euripides, Sappho, Shakespeare, Jefferson, Franklin, de Tocqueville, the various Adamses and Jameses, Douglass, Fuller, Dickinson, Whitman, Gilman, Wharton, Hemingway, Faulkner, Walker, King, and Morrison. Interestingly, many times the two "lists" overlap, as most public conversation also cites traditional authors.

To become culturally literate, of course, students need to know more than these writers' names, despite what the cultural lists compiled by William Bennett, Allan Bloom, and E.D. Hirsch seem to imply;[10] they need to know what these writers thought. The best way to accomplish this goal is to provide opportunities for students to engage these writers' ideas in their own texts (or in translation if the original is not in English)—to read the works, not what others say about the works. This activity would surely produce a reading list of great writers, great because of something significant they add to our knowledge of the human condition.

THE NECESSARY ADDITION

Perhaps the solution goes beyond the first-year English course. Since most first-year English courses focus primarily on communication, especially writing, and must also teach students to read, to view, to speak, and to think with critical awareness and, secondarily, to acquire some degree of computer literacy, the number of authors covered would necessarily be fairly limited. In order to accomplish the objective of producing students capable of understanding both literature and language, all students should also be required to take an upper-level literature class. This additional literature class would greatly broaden the range of authors available to all students. The proposed content change in the first-year courses to include studying authors who enable students to better understand the human condition would improve students' awareness of themselves and their world, and, thus, become an exercise in exploring what it means to be a humane and responsible person. The additional semester of literature would allow the process begun in that first year to continue.

However, the process can not stop there. The faculty of an institution must also participate in advocating works of authors they value to help students make the necessary connections. These proposed course content changes would allow students to engage texts that help them better understand themselves so that they, perhaps, will act thoughtfully and live as more humane, responsible, and productive members of a free society. We need not only to teach students how to read and think critically, but also to engage them in discussions of values and meaning. Then students will have a foundation from which to make better ethical decisions and responsible choices.

Again, in *On Moral Fiction*, Gardner recalls an old legend to illustrate just how difficult making the right choice can be. It seems that when Woden sought advice from the king of the trolls on what he must do to win the imminent battle with the enemies of order, the troll demanded that Woden give up his left eye as the price for the knowledge. After Woden willingly sacrificed his left eye because he was all too aware of what was at stake, he was told that the secret to success was to "Watch with both eyes!"[11] Perhaps before sacrificing the knowledge gained from literature for the "secrets" the new composition theories offer, it might be wise to consider how to use both.

Those who question this approach or the purpose and value of this kind of a liberal arts education might consider what a Boston University Center for Space Physics electrical engineer had to say when he appeared before the Massachusetts Board of Education to object to eliminating art, music, and physical education positions in order to buy computers: "The purpose of the schools [is] to, as one teacher argues, 'Teach carpentry, not [how to use a] hammer,'... . We need to teach the whys and ways of the world. Tools come and tools go. Teaching our children tools limits their knowledge to these tools and hence limits their futures."[12] Perhaps the best option is not either/or but rather to learn from Woden's mistake, and "Watch with both eyes." Certainly first-year English classes must serve the college and teach composition, but through the study of literature they must also help "students acquire knowledge and develop a critical awareness which allow them to live humanely, responsibly, and productively in a free society."[13]

NOTES

1. John Guillory, *Cultural Capital: The Problem of Literary Canon Formation* (Chicago: University of Chicago Press, 1993), 77-82.
2. A similar shift in values occurred in both England and in the United States during the late seventeenth and early eighteenth centuries, when the language of vernacular literature gradually replaced the classical languages as the elite language taught by the schools.
3. Quoted in Guillory, 80.
4. John Gardner, *On Moral Fiction* (New York: Basic Books, 1978), 5.
5. David Denby, *Great Books: My Adventures with Homer, Rousseau, Woolf, and Other Indestructible Writers of the Western World* (New York: Simon and Schuster, 1996), 459.
6. Harold Bloom, *The Western Canon: The Book and School of the Ages* (New York: Harcourt Brace, 1994), 30.
7. Although some readers operate under the mistaken notion that Plato banished poetry from his ideal city in *The Republic*, M.F. Burnyeat asserts, "Yes, he did banish Homer, Aeschylus, Sophocles, Euripides, Aristophanes – the greatest names of Greek literature. But not because they were poets. He banished them because they produced the wrong sort of poetry." What Plato denigrates is "false poetry," that which presents incorrect information about moral conduct, especially that of the gods. Instead of eliminating it, the right kind of poetry becomes almost omnipresent in his perfect but highly controlled society because Plato recognizes the power of poetry. In fact, he considers it so powerful that he will only permit the reading of the right kind of poetry, which served as the main source of information for Plato's Greeks.
8. In addition to Gardner, see also Matthew Arnold, *Culture and Anarchy*, ed. J. Dover Wilson (Cambridge: Cambridge University Press, 1932).
9. Dennis O'Brien, "The Disappearing Moral Curriculum," *The Key Reporter* 62.4 (1997): 4-5.
10. In all fairness, Hirsch's *Cultural Literacy* does contain some valuable explanatory information, but the list at the end does seem to suggest that if one is familiar with these people's names, then one has "cultural literacy."
11. Gardner, 3.
12. Todd Oppenheimer, "The Computer Delusion," *The Atlantic Monthly* (July 1997): 62.
13. *Greensboro College Academic Catalog* (1996-97), 8.

QUESTIONS FOR DISCUSSION

1. What might the oppressed have to offer in increasing our understanding of the human condition? Would their insights be different from those gained through reading the traditional canon?

2. Are multiculturalism and diversity the enemies of the traditional canon? Is the traditional canon the enemy of multiculturalism and diversity?

3. Do technology and diversity require us to sacrifice knowledge gained in literature? Why or why not?

4. How is setting the canon, as discussed by Hebert, different from the process in which a professor engages when designing a syllabus?

5. If all faculty are to determine the important works of literature, what role does the literature professor have in deciding what students read and study?

6. How does a professor decide whether a writer has something significant to say? How does a student decide?

7. Do fields other than literature help train people to think critically? If so, how and in what ways?

8. If students come to college not knowing the tradition and not being habitual readers, how can teaching non-user friendly readings entice them to engage in serious study of the canon?

9. Do canonical studies guarantee development of critical thinking?

WHAT MATTERS FOR GOOD GOVERNMENT?

Nancy M. McElveen

ABSTRACT

The question of "what matters for good government" is central to works ranging from Plato's *Republic* to Jean Bethke Elshtain's *Democracy on Trial*. In seventeenth-century France the question was taken up by the *moralistes*, a group of authors of brief maxims, sketches, portraits, or thoughts that present reflections on human nature and society. This paper examines the responses of three *moralistes* to the question of "what matters for good government." As tutors to princes, Bossuet and Fénelon attempt to shape the character of the future king by stressing the nature and necessity of moral virtue in an absolute monarchy. Eighteenth-century successor to the *moralistes*, Montesquieu invites readers to reflect on moral, political, and social character. Finally, contemporary political philosopher Elshtain maintains that modern civil society is likewise based on the ancient models of moral virtue.

Plato's *Republic* raises the question of who should rule in an ideal city. After describing the education of those who are to be called philosopher-kings, Socrates turns his attention to the institutions that will form them and the city where they will rule. He demands of Glaucon,

> Then who [*sic*] will you compel to become guardians of the city, if not those who have the best understanding of what matters for good government and who have other honors than political ones, and a better life as well? (*Republic* 521b)[1]

Centuries later, in seventeenth-century France, the question of "what matters for good government" was taken up by a group of writers at the court of Louis XIV. Known as *moralistes*, these writers were authors of brief maxims, sketches, portraits, or thoughts that present reflections on human nature and society.

This paper examines the responses of three *moralistes* to the question of "what matters for good government." Funeral orations delivered by court preacher and historiographer Jacques-Bénigne Bossuet not only eulogized their royal subjects, but they also essayed to caution the monarch, reminding him of the qualities essential to kingship. François de Salignac de la Mothe-Fénelon, heir to Bossuet's political theories, re-wrote the story of Telemachus, son of Ulysses, as a primer in kingship for the grandson of Louis XIV, preparing him for the day when he would inherit his grandfather's throne. The "Troglodyte Letters" of the *Persian Letters* of Charles-Louis de Secondat, baron de la Brède et de Montesquieu, show that this eighteenth-century successor to the *moralistes* must have carefully studied Fénelon's work.[2]

For the *moralistes*, as for Plato and Aristotle, "what matters for good government" calls into question whether governments are properly held to ethical standards of conduct, a question further divided into external relations (i.e., between governments) and internal ones (i.e., between a government and its people).[3] Both Plato and Aristotle concern themselves primarily with internal political relations, "with the extent to which the *polis* allows for the flourishing of its own citizen body."[4]

Plato's *Republic* constructs a model of a just state, one characterized by the existence of three social classes: workers and artisans, soldiers, and guardians. The guardian class, having excelled in education, will be chosen to undergo rigorous physical and intellectual training. The most capable among them, the philosophers, will be given complete political rule; a good ruler governs in virtue of the knowledge of truth: "For the state exists to guarantee the good life for its citizens and should thus be ruled by those with a developed capacity for approaching the essence of a good life...."[5]

Books VIII and IX of the *Republic* describe the degeneration of an "ideal philosophical aristocracy" into democracy and tyranny. Nevertheless, Plato affirms the responsibility of the *polis* to promote the good life for its citizens through education in virtue.[6]

In Aristotle's view, "The individual's good and the state's good are the same, but the state's attainment of the good is 'greater and more perfect' inasmuch as it means securing the good for the many."[7] The central moral category in Aristotle's ethical theory is virtue, defined as excellence. The "moral virtues" may be characterized as "excellences of the deliberative reason in its control of desires."[8]

Aristotle's *Nicomachean Ethics* presents the most complete form of social life as that of the *polis*: "Only in the *polis* can humans live the good life in its fullest sense...."[9] Monarchy, for Aristotle, is the ideal form of government, followed by aristocracy: "The polis exists for the positive advancement of commonly shared ideals of virtue and happiness, ..."[10]

Of these shared ideals Aristotle writes, "For even if the good is the same for the individual and the state, the good of the state is clearly the greater and more perfect thing to attain and to safeguard."[11]

Like Plato, Aristotle sees virtue in self-control and holds that moral virtue must be taught and learned:

> [W]e become just by the practice of just actions, self-controlled by exercising self-control, and courageous by performing acts of courage.
>
> This is corroborated by what happens in states. Lawgivers make the citizens good by inculcating (good) habits in them, and this is the aim of every lawgiver; if he does not succeed in doing that, his legislation is a failure (*Ethics* 1103a-1103b).

Like Plato and Aristotle, the French *moraliste*s held that moral virtue must be taught and learned. One form of training for virtue in seventeenth-century France was the education of the monarch, often by court-appointed tutors or other courtiers. The works of Bossuet, Fénelon, and Montesquieu all describe the role of virtue in "what matters for good government" when that government takes the form of absolute monarchy.

JACQUES-BENIGNE BOSSUET (1627-1704)

Orator, churchman, political thinker, and historian, Jacques-Bénigne Bossuet studied first at the Jesuit *collège* in Dijon, then completed his humanist education at the Collège de Navarre in Paris. Significantly, Bossuet's Jesuit education glorified the civic responsibility and republican spirit of ancient Rome and of the ancient Greeks.

THE *DISCOURSE ON UNIVERSAL HISTORY* AND THE *POLITICS*

In 1670 Bossuet was appointed as tutor to the Dauphin, the heir to the throne of Louis XIV. He developed for his royal pupil a theory of history which emphasized the role of Divine Providence in human affairs, a theory set forth in the *Discours sur l'histoire universelle* (*Discourse on Universal History*, 1681). However, Bossuet is best known for the *Politique tirée des propres paroles de l'Ecriture sainte* (*Politics as Taken from the Very Words of the Holy Scripture*, 1709), prepared for posthumous publication by the author's nephew, the abbé Bossuet. This ten-book treatise presents the most complete French statement of the theory of absolute monarchy and the divine right of kings. Bossuet's goal in writing the *Politique* was to give to the future king some sound principles:

> The *Politique* demands a king who is hardworking, scrupulous, attentive, careful to be well-informed and careful to consult the best advisors, but at the same time energetic and able to make his own decisions clearly and decisively.[12]

In Bossuet's view, the king should be brought up respecting the law in order to avoid becoming a tyrant.

Bossuet's primary concern is the foundation of legitimate power. In the *Politique* Bossuet affirms the superiority of hereditary monarchy over all other forms of government. He further affirms that all power comes from God. As Richard Lockwood points out,

> When he confronts the question of foundations and their reproduction or representation, Bossuet's invariable approach is to view authority in terms of descent or filiation. In chronological terms, legitimate authority is handed down through the ages, ...Synchronically, God invests power in his representatives, who rule over his people in the same way he rules over them.... Authority is vested in a single subject, who is an imitation of God, an example to the people, a sign, representing and making present the unity and omnipotence of God.[13]

While Bossuet affirms the right to individual liberty, he repeatedly stresses that the state's ultimate purpose is to render life pleasant and its people happy—a purpose stated in the *Discours sur l'histoire universelle* and echoed in the *Politique*.[14] The image of a happy people is offered by Bossuet to the sovereign, and it is that image which should direct the sovereign's preoccupations.[15]

Bossuet and his contemporaries envisioned the role of the king and his subject as like that of a shepherd and his flock, an image rooted in Biblical and patristic tradition. Another image of the king was that of father to his children. In one of his sermons as Bishop of Metz, Bossuet clearly defines royal authority as essentially paternal:

> It is a universal power to do good toward submissive peoples in such a way that the name of the king is like that of an ordinary father and general benefactor, and there lies the ray of divinity which shines forth in all sovereigns.[16]

For Bossuet and his contemporaries, the relationship between a sovereign and his people should therefore take place within the dual framework of the mystical body of the civil community (likened to the mystical body of the church), or *polis*, and the love of a father for his sons. And just as the king exhibits a paternal attitude toward his subjects, so in the Christian tradition must he display a filial attitude toward God. Only then can a prince be worthy of his title:

> The entire Christian tradition makes princes the privileged sons of God, and they ought to conform strictly to his teaching. The prince can only be worthy of his name when he reproduces in himself God's wisdom and imitates in his thoughts and acts the thoughts and acts of Jesus Christ.[17]

Throughout the *Politique*, Bossuet's goal is to closely unite his prince with God, thereby making him a faithful servant.[18] In the Fifth Book of the *Politique*, Bossuet writes, "God is holiness itself, goodness itself, power itself, reason itself. In these things is God's majesty. In the image of these things is the majesty of the prince."[19] Again Bossuet defines majesty as God's grandeur reflected in the prince ("La majesté est l'image de la grandeur de Dieu dans le prince" [177]).

As God cares for his flock, so the prince cares for his people, putting public welfare above all else: "The prince, as a prince, is not looked upon as a private man: he is a public figure, the whole state is within him, the will of all people is contained within his will."[20]

These themes of the *Politique*—the divine nature of the king and his concern for the welfare of his people—emerge as important themes in several of the funeral sermons preached by Bossuet. A brief examination of the *Oraisons funèbres* of Henriette de France, the Prince de Condé, and Marie-Thérèse d'Autriche reveals those lessons for the king.

THE FUNERAL SERMONS

Henriette d'Angleterre. Henriette de France (1609-1669), the youngest child of Henri IV and Marie de Médicis, was married at the age of sixteen to the Protestant King Charles I of England. Pope Urban VIII permitted their mixed-religion marriage in the hope of bringing religious unity to England. When uprisings began against the king, Henriette fought valiantly in defense of the crown. Seeking refuge in 1644, Henriette returned to Paris, where she was given a royal welcome. However, during the 1648 revolt of the nobles known as the Fronde, Prime Minister Mazarin prevented payment of her pension. Despite having endured all manner of misfortune, Henriette saw her family rise again. Her son Charles II was restored to his father's throne, and her daughter Henriette married the duc d'Orléans, brother of Louis XIV. Henriette ended her life quietly in the convent of Chaillot in Paris, where she died on November 10, 1669, at the age of sixty. At the request of Madame la duchesse d'Orléans, Henriette's daughter, Bossuet agreed to pronounce her funeral oration.

Bossuet begins his *Oraison funèbre* for Henriette d'Angleterre by portraying first the queen's grandeur, then her misfortune. Throughout the *Oraison funèbre* the queen's virtues are self-evident: courage in times of struggle, clemency in victory, resignation in defeat, and unwavering piety toward the God who had made her an unhappy queen. Early in the funeral sermon, Bossuet reminds the mourners that kings are made, elevated, or defeated by God:

> He who reigns in the heavens and on whom all empires depend, to whom alone belong glory, majesty, and independence, he alone also glorifies himself and his majesty to kings and gives to them, as it pleases him, grand and terrible lessons.[21]

Indeed, according to Bossuet, earthly kings have only borrowed majesty (112). The life of Henriette, retold in her funeral sermon, should be an example to future rulers, who should learn from her just as she had learned from God:

> But the wise and devout princess who is the subject of this sermon was not only a spectacle presented to men for studying the counsels of Divine Providence and the fatal revolutions of monarchies, she herself was instructed, while God was instructing princes by her example.[22]

In all circumstances, Henriette was a model of virtue, always kind and pleasant but strong and steadfast, prudent in all dealings and magnanimous.[23] Indeed, Henriette exemplified the duties of kings as they were prescribed by Pope Gregory:

> Sovereign power is granted to you from on high so that virtue might be assisted, that the paths to Heaven might be widened, and so that the earthly empire might serve the empire of Heaven.[24]

For Bossuet, the most suitable use of power is to aid virtue and to uphold right (117).[25]

Having recounted the misfortunes of Henriette, Bossuet returns to one of the central themes of his sermon, the reminder that the first responsibility of a ruler is the welfare of his people. Bossuet explains that a prince who pursues only his own interests and gives himself over to excess risks causing great harm to his people:

> One finds that up to now that they [great changes] have been caused either by the softness of the violence of princes. Indeed, when princes, neglecting to recognize their affairs and their armies, working only at hunting, having glory only for luxuriousness, having wit only to invent pleasures; or, when carried away by their violent humour, they keep neither laws nor measures, and they dare both the respect and the fear of men, by making the ills that they suffer even more intolerable than those that they foresee: thus either excessive license or patience pushed to the extreme threatens terribly the ruling houses.[26]

Another major theme of the *Oraison funèbre* of Henriette d'Angleterre is a plea for religious unity, an end to the multiple Protestant sects, and a desire to reunite all peoples in the Catholic Church. In this endeavor princes should lead by example, putting aside their own self-interest for that of the people they serve,[27] as Plato's philosopher-kings were instructed to do.

Finally, Bossuet reminds his hearers of the consequences of excess: "Great prosperities blind us, transport us, cause us to forget God, ourselves, and the sentiments of faith. Thence are born monsters, crimes, refinements of pleasure,..."[28] Like Plato, Bossuet prescribes royal restraint, even to the point of austerity. Bossuet concludes this sermon with a reminder of Henriette's courage and patience through long years of adversity, virtues rewarded by the accession to the English throne of her son Charles II and a restoration of the family's good name. The memory of Henriette d'Angleterre will stand as a reminder of the lessons of faith of Bossuet's *Discours sur l'histoire universelle*: God uses catastrophes to draw his people back into the fold.[29]

Marie-Thérèse d'Autriche. A similar message concerning the importance of faith is the central lesson of the *Oraison funèbre* of Marie-Thérèse d'Autriche, wife of Louis XIV. Marie-Thérèse was born in 1638 to Philip IV of Spain and his wife, Isabelle de Bourbon, daughter of Henri IV of France. Her mother died when Marie-Thérèse was six years old; the child lived in her father's court until negotiations between France and Spain culminated in the Treaty of the Pyrenees in 1659. One of the principal terms of the treaty was the marriage of

Marie-Thérèse to Louis XIV. As queen of France, Marie-Thérèse had no power and no influence in the business of the kingdom. Indeed, she had neither a taste nor a talent for political affairs. She gave birth to six children, five of whom died.

Marie-Thérèse suffered the loss of her children, as well as the king's misconduct and her subsequent abandonment. Nevertheless, she found courage and resignation in her ardent piety and exemplary charity. Before her death, Marie-Thérèse saw the king return to her and correct the excesses of his private life.

Faced with the problem of what to say about a queen who took so little part in court life and in the events of her time, Bossuet associated her with the king and the glories of his reign. In the *Oraison funèbre* of Marie-Thérèse, Bossuet praised her unswerving faith, her visible practice of piety, and her love for the sacraments of the Church, especially the Eucharist.

Bossuet began his funeral sermon by praising the royal houses of France and Austria. In the tradition of the *Discours universelle*, Bossuet places the queen in the plan of Divine Providence, noting that God had placed Marie-Thérèse at the summit of human greatness in order to present her as a model for all mankind:

> God raised her to the height of human grandeurs in order to render more striking and more exemplary the purity and perpetual conformity of her life. Thus, her life and her death, equally filled with holiness and grace, become instruction for the human race.[30]

Above all, Marie-Thérèse was a model of constant virtue, and Bossuet urges the assembled mourners to hasten to contemplate her example: "Run, peoples: come to contemplate, in the first place in the world, the rare and majestic beauty of an ever-constant virtue."[31]

Having situated the queen securely in the lineage of the French royal house, Bossuet emphasizes that by both her virtuous upbringing and her birth Marie-Thérèse was worthy of and destined for Louis XIV:

> All of the most virtuous and clever things of Spain were brought around her. She saw herself, so to speak, completely surrounded by virtues, and there appeared in this young princess more beautiful qualities than she expected in crowns. Philip thus raised her for his States; God, who loves us, destined her for Louis.[32]

Throughout the sermon Bossuet praises Marie-Thérèse as the ideal, divinely-appointed consort for Louis XIV. Her constant piety and devotion had tempered the excesses of the king. Under her influence, Louis had become a model king, like those of the Old Testament, according to the plan of Divine Providence. Having praised the queen's dignity and her deep faith, made visible by her observances of the sacraments, Bossuet exhorts the courtiers to learn from her example: "You will learn from the Queen how to preserve such purity in this place of temptations and among the world's illusions of grandeur."[33]

He repeatedly stresses not only the virtues of Marie-Thérèse, but also in the ways in which her piety supports the king, who shares his glory with her:

> [W]hat I repeat with admiration [is] that the inexplicable tenderness of Marie-Thérèse tended to inspire in him faith, piety, the fear of God, an inviolable attachment to the king, mercy for the unfortunate, an unchanging perseverance in all his duties, and all that we praise in this prince's conduct.[34]

The Prince de Condé. As he had done in the *Oraison funèbre* of Marie-Thérèse, Bossuet intends to instruct the hearers of the funeral sermon for the Prince de Condé about the importance of piety and devotion, qualities which take precedence over courage and intelligence ("les qualités du coeur et de l'esprit" [1328]). Bossuet preached the funeral sermon of his longtime friend at the request of the king.

Louis Bourbon II, prince de Condé (1621-1686) was known as "le Grand Condé"; after his father's death in 1646, he became known as Monsieur le Prince. Condé was a brilliant student at the Jesuit *collège* in Bourges. He married a niece of Richelieu and joined the army at the age of nineteen. When he was barely twenty-two, Condé was made commander-in-chief of troops assigned to push Spanish troops back from the northern borders of France. As the victor in the 1643 Battle of Rocroi against Spain, Condé came into conflict with the royalists in the Fronde. In his retirement at Chantilly Condé was a major patron of artists and writers, among them Boileau, Racine, and La Bruyère.

Condé died on December 11, 1686, and Bossuet preached his funeral sermon at Notre Dame in Paris on March 10, 1687. In the *Oraison funèbre*, Bossuet—who also held the post of royal historiographer—speaks as a well-informed and impartial historian, retracing Condé's career. He tells the truth about Condé, including his faults. Bossuet is quite emphatic about the transitory nature of earthly glory, reminding his audience that glory which is not founded upon a solid base of piety is for naught: "All that glory would be nothing if it did not rest on a more solid base."[35] Indeed, the power of the nothing if it did not rest on a more solid base."[35] Indeed, the power of the conquering general—just like that of the monarch—comes directly from God: "Without this inestimable gift of piety, what would the prince de Condé be [even] with all this great courage and great genius!"[36]

For Condé, just as for other royal personages eulogized by Bossuet, the ultimate objective of all his actions was to do good and to seek virtue before glory: "Indeed, he had as a principle ...that in great deeds he must think only of doing good and to allow glory to come after virtue."[37] Whatever glory Condé achieved was employed in the king's service and for the good of the state: "[E]verything tended toward the true and the great. Thence it came that he put his glory in the service of the king and in the happiness of the state:...."[38]

After praising Condé as a sort of Renaissance man, Bossuet cautions against worldly vanity, reminding his hearers once again of the source of their greatness: "O kings, reduce yourselves to silence in your grandeur; conquerors, do not boast of your victories."[39]

As Bossuet concludes his oration, he reminds the mourners that Condé was not only a military hero; he was also an exemplary father:

> These are simple things, to govern his family, to educate his domestic servants, to show justice and mercy, to accomplish the good which God wishes, these are the common practices of the Christian life that Jesus Christ will praise at the last day before his holy angels and before his heavenly Father.[40]

FRANÇOIS DE SALIGNAC DE LA MOTHE-FÉNELON (1651-1715)

Heir to Bossuet's notion of a *Providence particulière* that had furnished David and Solomon to ancient Israel and Louis XIV to France, François de Salignac de la Mothe-Fénelon (1651-1715) was born to a noble but impoverished family in the Périgord, a region in the southwest of France. Educated for the Church first by the Jesuits in Cahors, then at St-Sulpice in Paris, Fénelon was ordained in the priesthood in 1675 and received into the Académie Française in 1693. Fénelon went to live with his uncle Antoine, marquis de Fénelon, at the abbey of St-Germain-des-Prés, where he met Bossuet.[41]

In 1689 Fénelon was named as tutor to the duc de Bourgogne, grandson of Louis XIV. Banished from the court in 1697,[42] Fénelon was divested of both his pension and his position as tutor in 1699. The premature death of the prince in 1712 marked the end of Fénelon's hopes for a renewed France. Fénelon himself never returned to Versailles or to Paris and died in January 1715.

Although directed by Bossuet, the education of the young prince's father, the Dauphin, had been a dismal failure, characterized by boredom, constraint, and cruelty. In Fénelon's mind, the Duke's lessons should fit the needs of kingship. Pedantry was to be replaced by an atmosphere that was intimate, pleasurable, and paternal. Thus Fénelon began to write original compositions which would convey to the young prince basic lessons in conduct and morality. In a general sense, Fénelon advocates the adoption of a moral code, "the touchstone of which is an all-embracing concept of virtue."[43] For Fénelon, the education of the prince is an affair of State; the reward for his success is the happiness of the people.

In the *Dialogues des morts, composés pour l'éducation d'un prince*, composed in 1692-93, leading figures from both antiquity and modern times converse on power, corruption, destiny, vanity, and human ambition. Fénelon's aim in the *Dialogues des morts* was to show the duc de Bourgogne what he might become, should he forget the wise counsel of his youth.[44]

THE ADVENTURES OF TELEMACHUS

Sometime between 1694 and 1696, Fénelon composed what remains his best-known work, *Les Aventures de Télémaque, fils d'Ulysse* (*The Adventures of Telemachus, Son of Ulysses*).[45] At its publication, *Telemachus* was considered a harsh personal critique of the reign of Louis XIV. Fénelon was born in the year that Louis XIV attained his majority. By the time Fénelon entered court circles, the panoply of splendor and power that characterized the court of the Sun King had begun to reveal social, moral, and political decay. Fénelon reveals himself as an adversary of war, luxury, and absolutism. Fénelon's use of the form of an heroic epic in an ancient setting corresponds in many ways to the use of historical or mythological subjects by the playwrights of the classical theater. By setting his tale in a time and place far removed from the court of Louis XIV, Fénelon could avoid at least the appearance of direct criticism of the reigning monarch. Early in the narrative, Telemachus tells Calypso of being instructed by his companion Mentor in the tales of gods and heroes:[46]

> They proceeded then to talk of the origin of the gods, of heroes, of poets, the golden age, the deluge, the first histories of mankind, the river of oblivion in

the impious in the black gulf of Tartarus, and that happy peace which the just enjoy in the Elysian Fields without any fear of forfeiting.[47]

Nevertheless, the court saw Louis XIV in the figure of Idomeneus, the luxury-loving king given over to waging war and to enjoying pleasure. To the court, Telemachus clearly represented the duc de Bourgogne, and Fénelon himself was Mentor.[48]

Why should Fénelon choose Telemachus as the hero of his story of the "moral and political education of a young man by a knowledgeable and virtuous tutor" [49]? Telemachus, who providentially vanishes from Book 5 to Book 15 of the *Odyssey*, is young and not fully formed. Besides, he is the son of Ulysses, the wisest of the heroes of the Trojan War, and he is destined to be king of Ithaca.[50]

Fénelon's novel, divided into eighteen books, begins when Telemachus and Mentor are shipwrecked on the isle of the goddess Calypso, who warmly welcomes the son of Ulysses. Calypso tells Telemachus of his father's adventures, offers him immortality (which he refuses just as his father had done), and begs him to tell her of his own adventures. As the adventures of Telemachus unfold, Fénelon reveals his political stance and the political realities of the day, his notions of the monarchy, and the role of the king's virtue in governing his people. Although he situates his story in antiquity, Fénelon clearly aims to influence the present, not to explain the past. *Telemachus* is above all a pedagogical work, written for a young man destined to be king, not a program of government. Fénelon's project was to make his royal pupil aware of the difficulties he would confront when he began to rule, to call to his attention the huge stakes—no less than the future of his pupil's kingdom—and to furnish the tools and the criteria for analysis and judgment, not to suggest solutions to all the problems which France was facing at the end of the reign of Louis XIV.[51]

Fénelon reveals himself as a traditionalist, a partisan of inherited divine-right monarchy. Nevertheless, as Fénelon joins in the fundamental debate about the role of the individual in society, his position is clear: the common good is more important than the welfare of a single individual.[52] Like Bossuet, Fénelon is firmly convinced that the sole purpose of government—and hence the duty of the king—is to make the people happy.

Partisan though he is, Fénelon points out the dangers of absolutism, even as he attempts to demonstrate that it is a form of government that requires wisdom, patience, and justice in its administration. He insists that the king has absolute power to do good for his people, and that the king's power to harm his people should be limited by law. In response to Telemachus's questions about people should be limited by law. In response to Telemachus's questions about the extent of the king's authority, Mentor explains, "He can do anything to the people; but the laws can do anything to him. He has an absolute power in doing good, but his hands are tied from doing wrong (60)."[53] Indeed, this obedience to the law distinguishes the tyrant from the legitimate ruler, educated in virtue.[54]

While Bossuet had offered a defense of divine-right monarchy based on a claim that the rule of Louis XIV had descended in an unbroken line from Abraham's covenant in Genesis, Fénelon theorized a "republican" monarchy, whose key traits included simplicity, the absence of luxury and splendor, and the elevation of peace over war and aggrandizement. Throughout more than half of the eighteen books, Telemachus is exposed, either through direct instruction or through observation, to principles which should guide a wise and virtuous monarch. Among those principles were the necessity for the king to love his subjects and to expend his energy in the pursuit of their welfare; the necessity for the king to be surrounded by capable, sincere advisors and to be immune to flattery; and the necessity for the king to set an example of simple, frugal, unostentatious living. As Telemachus recounts his adventures to Calypso, he tells of his treatment at the hands of Metophis, an officer of the court of Sesostris, king of Thebes. Quickly Telemachus learned that kings are often exposed to misrepresentations; even the wisest are deceived: "Hélas! À quoi les rois sont-ils exposés! Les plus sages mêmes sont souvent surpris" (87).

As advisor to Idomeneus—and as an example to Telemachus—Mentor counseled reduction of the pomp and luxury that tend to corrupt a people. He recommended reducing everything to a state of frugality and simplicity: food and drink, music, architecture, and clothing and ornament. Mentor reminded Idomeneus that he must set an example for his people:

> 'I know of but one way,' he said to Idomeneus, 'to prevent frugality from falling into disgrace among your people; and that is by setting an example of it yourself.' ...the sage Mentor satisfied him that these laws, though revived, would signify nothing unless he enforced them by his own example, which could alone give them authority (162, 163-64).[55]

Another essential element of a virtuous king's domestic policy, according to Fénelon, was the maintenance of moral order. The king should watch over the education of his people. He should see that schools are established in which the young people are taught to fear the gods, to love their country, to respect the laws, and to prefer honor to pleasure or even to life itself.[56]

On the foreign policy front, Fénelon condemns war, especially wars of conquest; such wars bring only disgrace to the human race and false glory to the king who seeks to acquire glory by war:

> War is sometimes necessary, it is true; but it is the shame of the human race, though it should be inevitable on certain occasions. O kings, do not say at all that one should desire to acquire glory: true glory is not found at all outside of humanity.[57]

Nevertheless, a nation might be called upon to defend itself; therefore, it is appropriate to be prepared for war. Mentor urges Telemachus to join the young men of Crete in the army, so that they should not be ignorant of the art of war:

> [B]ut, lest the whole nation should sink into effeminacy, and ignorance of the art of war, it is proper that the young nobility should be sent to the wars abroad. These will be sufficient to keep up the whole nation in an emulation for glory, in the love of arms, in a contempt of hardship and death itself, and in experience of military art (154).[58]

CHARLES-LOUIS DE SECONDAT BARON DE LA BRÈDE ET DE MONTESQUIEU (1689-1755)

Fénelon's *Télémaque* would have lasting political and moral effects on pre-Enlightenment and Enlightenment writers. Patrick Riley points out that

> The troglodytes of Montesquieu's *Lettres persanes* (*Persian Letters*) of 1721 recall those noble savages of La Bétique [one of the kingdoms visited by Telemachus and Mentor], and his views on the efficacy of laws in *L'Esprit des lois* (*The Spirit of the Laws*) indicate that he must have carefully studied Fénelon's romance.[59]

Published anonymously (probably in Amsterdam) in 1721, the *Persian Letters* purports to tell the tale of two travelers, Usbek and Rica, who set out from Persia to visit France. In their letters the travelers comment on French institutions and on French life as they find it.

Montesquieu presents, in the person of Usbek, the portrait of a despot. In contrast, in letters 11-14, he tells the story of the Troglodytes, illustrating the fall of a *polis* ruled by self-interest and its subsequent renaissance in an atmosphere where the common good prevailed over individual concerns. The allegorical story of the Troglodytes, inspired by Fénelon and by the Greek historian Herodotus, begins as Usbek describes a people living in a primitive state, people who resembled beasts more than human beings.[60] Their principle industry was agriculture, and they only used simple, practical arts. Their king, who was of foreign origin, set out to correct their vicious nature ("la méchanceté de leur naturel"[53]) by treating them severely. But the people plotted against the king and killed him and all his family. After much dissension, the Troglodytes elected magistrates as their new rulers. But the magistrates proved equally intolerable, and the people massacred them too. They thus decided to live a life of selfishness ("que chacun veillerait uniquement à ses intérêts, sans consulter ceux des autres" [54]). That life ultimately led to the destruction of the Troglodytes. In the second part of the allegory, Montesquieu presents two Troglodyte families who were different by nature from the others. They were naturally virtuous ("[I]ls avaient de l'humanité; ils connaissaient la justice; ils aimaient la vertu" [57]). They worked together, with care for the common good ("[I]ls travaillaient avec une sollicitude commune pour l'intérêt commun" [57]). The virtuous Troglodytes triumphed over their enemies and ultimately agreed to choose a king. However, the most just man among them took the crown with much reluctance.

The tale of the Troglodytes invites readers to reflect on moral, political, and social character. Convinced that laws are the basis for the mores of a nation, Montesquieu wished to denounce the danger posed to the French nation by despotism and intolerance. Behind the oriental fiction of the *Persian Letters* lie two lessons which Montesquieu would develop in the *Spirit of the Laws*: despotism corrupts unceasingly because it is corrupt by nature, and despotism causes terrible evil to human nature.

The writings of Bossuet, Fénelon, and Montesquieu argue that a society's political institutions have power of determination over the moral life and happiness of individuals. Their power was accompanied by responsibility for the welfare of citizens and for their morals.[61] For men of the eighteenth century, as for Aristotle, politics and ethics were inseparable. Happiness, virtue, and the reconciliation of public and private interest were constant goals of both politics and ethics. As the eighteenth century progressed, two major patterns of thought emerged:

> One held that government has the power and the duty to change the modes of behavior, feeling, and thinking of the individual. The other limited the function of government to the administrative regulation of the mechanisms of the State, the equitable adjustment of conflicts of interest, and protection of individual rights.[62]

MODERN DEMOCRATIC SOCIETY

As the events of the eighteenth century unfolded, cultural transformation redefined the roles of men as would-be citizens of a harmonious polity, purifying public, social, and political institutions which affected them. Thirty years before the French Revolution, Jean-Jacques Rousseau wrote that the "general will ...is the rule of justice agreed upon by assemblies of free people whose interest is only to serve the welfare of the society and of each person in it."[63] In her *Meditations on Modern Political Thought*, Jean Bethke Elshtain describes Rousseau as the father of civic republicanism; she writes,

> For Rousseau, to be a citizen is to undergo a dramatic civic transformation.... The man-become-citizen gives himself to the polity and internalizes an absolutely binding civic religion with demanding articles of faith.[64]

For the rulers addressed by Bossuet and Fénelon, and for the man-become-citizen of Montesquieu and Rousseau, civic virtues included frugality, simplicity, and concern for the common good. Modern democratic society has likewise assumed such civic virtues in its citizens. Writing about the precarious state of American democracy, Elshtain maintains that

> Civil society is a realm that is neither individualist nor collectivist.... The Anti-Federalists ...pushed an idealized image of a self-reliant republic that shunned imperial power and worked, instead, to create a polity modeled on classic principles of civic virtue and the common good.[65]

Confronted by scandal-ridden government at all levels, contemporary American society appears to be divided in its concept of what matters for good government. On the one hand are those who see their leaders in the patristic, if not exactly Biblical, role held by the kings of early modern France. Citizens who hold that view consider that their father-figure leaders should be models of virtue, above reproach. On the other hand are those who consider their leaders to be among the ranks of common men, with faults and foibles just like their own. Engaging in a *laissez-faire* approach to leadership, these citizens are content to let their leaders live as they will, as long as their lifestyles do not appear to interfere with their ability to govern effectively. In order to allow good government to persist, this dichotomy must be resolved. As in Plato's hypothetical society, it is the responsibility of the *polis* to promote the good life for its citizens through education in virtue. Moral and civic virtue, including justice, self-control, and courage, must be continuously taught and learned. In contemporary American democracy, just as in the absolute monarchy that monarchy that occupied the thought of Bossuet and Fénelon, the leader's first responsibility must be the welfare of the people. The contemporary leader who pursues his own interests or yields to his own excesses risks causing great harm to his people, just as Plato, Aristotle, and the *moralistes* had cautioned centuries before.

The monarch of Bossuet and his contemporaries was heir to the medieval notion of the king's two bodies. The king's public persona was separate and wholly distinct from his private person. The relationship between the king and his subjects existed on the level of the public, official persona. The king's private person did not enter into the arena of government. But in contemporary American society, the relationship between the leader and the people must take place within the dual framework of the civil community and the paternal concern of the leader for the citizens. The leader of a contemporary democracy is not a private individual; he is a public figure who carries the whole state and the collective will of the people within him. In contemporary society, just as in the societies envisioned by Plato and Aristotle, it is the individual virtue of the leader that gives rise to good public governance.

NOTES

1. Plato, *Republic*, trans. G.M.A. Grube, rev. C.D.C. Reeve (Indianapolis: Hackett Publishing Co., 1992). All quotations are from this edition and will be cited by parenthetical references in the text.
2. James Herbert Davis, Jr., *Fénelon* (Boston: Twayne Publishers, 1979), 109.
3. John E. Hare, "Ethics in Government," *Encyclopedia of Ethics*, Vol. I (New York: Garland Publishing Inc., 1992), 412.
4. *Encyclopedia of Ethics,* Vol. I, 413.
5. James B. Tubbs, Jr. & James F. Childress, "Platonic Ethics," *Westminster Dictionary of Christian Ethics* (Philadelphia: Westminster Press, 1986), 478.
6. "Platonic Ethics," 478.
7. Tubbs & Childress, "Aristotelian Ethics," *Westminster Dictionary of Christian Ethics*, 39.
8. "Aristotelian Ethics," 41.
9. Ibid., 41.
10. Ibid., 41.

11. Aristotle, *Nicomachaean Ethics*, trans. Martin Ostwald. Library of Liberal Arts (Englewood Cliffs, NJ: Prentice-Hall, 1962), 1094b. All quotations from the *Ethics* are from this edition and will be cited parenthetically in the text.

12. Jacques Truchet, ed., *Politique de Bossuet* (Paris: Armand Colin, 1966), 40. "La *Politique* exige un roi laborieux, scrupuleux, attentif, soucieux de s'informer et de consulter les meilleurs conseillers, mais énergique et sachant prendre ses décisions seul et avec netteté." All translations are mine unless otherwise indicated.

13. Richard Lockwood, "Figures of Power: Rhetoric and Political Theory in Bossuet," *Cahiers du dix-septième* (Spring 1992), 129.

14. Jacques-Bénigne Bossuet, *La Politique tirée des propres paroles de l'Ecriture sainte*, ed. Jacques LeBrun (Genève: Droz, 1967), xxix. All citations from the *Politique* are from this edition and will be noted by page number.

15. Bossuet, in the *Politique*, echoes the work of the Jesuit St. Robert Bellarmine (1542-1621), archbishop of Capua and later a cardinal. According to Bellarmine,

> [C]elui auquel le gouvernement des autres est commis, les surpasse aussi bien in vertu qu'en puissance et que sa vie n'étant souillée d'aucune tâche, reluise par l'éclat de toutes les perfections qui doivent être inséparables du reste des monarques. [The one to whom is entrusted the government of others should surpass them as much in virtue as in power, and, his life unsoiled by any blot, he should shine from all those perfections which ought to be inseparable from other monarchs.] (Bellarmine, "De officio principis christiani," Rome, 1619). Cited by Raymond Darricau, "Princes et peuples dans leur réciproque fidélité chez les docteurs catholiques de Bellarmine à Muratori," in Yves Durand, ed., *Hommages à Roland Mousnier: Clientèles et fidélités en Europe à l'Epoque moderne* [Paris: Presses Universitaires de France, 1981]), 29-30.

16. Bossuet, *IIe Sermon pour la circoncision*, à Metz, vers 1656. Cited in Darricau, 36.

> C'est une puissance universelle de faire du bien aux peuples soumis: tellement que le nom de roi, c'est un nom commun et de bienfaiteur général; et c'est là ce rayon de divinité que éclate dans les souverains.

17. Darricau, 40.

> Toute la tradition chrétienne fait des princes les fils privilégiés de Dieu qui doivent conformer étroitement leur vie à son enseignement. Le prince ne peut être vraiment digne de son nom que s'il reproduit en lui la sagesse de Dieu et imite dans ses pensées et dans ses actes les pensées et les actes de Jésus-Christ.

18. Darricau, 41.

19. "Dieu est la sainteté même, la bonté même, la puissance même, la raison même. En l'image de ces choses est la majesté du prince" (79).

20. "Le prince, en tant que prince, n'est pas regardé comme un homme particulier: c'est un personnage public, tout l'Etat est en lui, la volonté de tout le peuple est renfermée dans la sienne" (177-178).

21. Bossuet, *Oeuvres*, ed. L'Abbé Velat & Yvonne Champailler (Paris: Gallimard, 1961), 111. All citations from the *Oraisons funèbres* are from this edition; for further references, page numbers will be noted in the text.

> Celui qui règne dans les cieux, et de qui relèvent tous les empires, à qui seul appartient la gloire, la majesté, et l'indépendance, et aussi qui se glorifie de faire la lui aux rois, et de leur donner, quand il lui plaît, de grandes et de terribles leçons.

22. "Mais la sage et religieuse princesse qui fait le sujet de ce discours n'a pas été seulement un spectacle proposé aux hommes pour y étudier les conseils de la divine Providence, et les fatales révolutions des monarchies; elle s'est instruit elle-même, pendant que Dieu instruisait les princes par son exemple" (113).

23. "Douce, familière, agréable autant que ferme et vigoureuse, elle savait persuader et convaincre aussi bien que commander, et faire valoir la raison non moins que l'autorité. Vous verrez avec quelle prudence elle traitait les affaires, ...On ne peut assez louer la magnanimité de cette princesse." [Kind, familiar, pleasant, as well as firm and vigorous, she knows how to persuade and convince as well as to command, and to make reason valued no less than authority. You will see how prudently she conducted things, ...One cannot praise enough the magnanimity of this princess" (113).

24. "[L]a souveraine puissance vous êtes accordée d'en haut afin que la vertu soit aidée, que les voies du Ciel soient élargies et que l'empire de la terre serve l'empire du Ciel" (117).

25. "Car qu'y a-t-il de plus convenable à la puissance que de secourir la vertu? À quoi la force doit-elle servir, qu'à défendre la raison?" [What is more powerful than to aid virtue? For what should might serve but to defend the right?].

26. *Oeuvres*, 122.

> [O]n trouve que jusques ici elles [les grandes mutations] sont causées, ou par la mollesse, ou par la violence des princes. En effet, quand les princes, négligeant de connaître leurs affaires et leurs armées, ne travaillent qu'à la chasse, ...n'ont de gloire que pour le luxe, ni d'esprit que pour inventer des plaisirs; ou quand, emportés par leur humeur violente, ils ne gardent plus ni lois ni mesures, et qu'ils ôtent les égards et la crainte aux hommes, en faisant que les maux qu'ils souffrent leur paraissent plus insupportables que ceux qu'ils prévoient: alors ou la licence excessive, ou la patience poussée à l'extrémité, menacent terriblement les maisons régnantes.

27. *Oeuvres*, 126, 130. "Les sujets ont cessé d'en révérer les maximes quand ils les ont vus céder aux passions et aux intérêts de leurs princes" (126). "C'était le conseil de Dieu d'instruire les rois à ne point quitter son Eglise" (130) [Subjects have ceased to revere its maxims when they have seen them yield to the passions and [self-]interests of their princes...It was God's counsel to instruct kings that they should never leave his Church].

28. "Les grandes prospérités nous aveuglent, nous transportent, nous égarent, nous font oublier Dieu, nous-mêmes, et les sentiments de la foi. De là naissent des monstres, des crimes, des raffinements de plaisir (140).

29. "Puisse-t-il la placer au sein d'Abraham et, content de ses maux, épargner désormais à sa famille at au monde de si terribles leçons?" [Might one place her in the bosom of Abraham, and, content with her misfortunes, spare her family and the world from such terrible lessons?] (143).

30. "Dieu l'a élevée au faîte des grandeurs humaines, afin de rendre la pureté et la perpétuelle régularité de sa vie plus éclatante et plus exemplaire. Ainsi sa vie et sa mort, également pleines de sainteté et de grâce, deviennent l'instruction du genre humain" (208).

31. "Accourez, peuples: venez contempler dans la première place du monde la rare et majestueuse beauté d'une vertu toujours constante" (212).

32. "[O]n approcha d'elle tout ce que l'Espagne avait de plus vertueux et de plus habile. Elle se vit, pour ainsi parler, dès son enfance, tout environnée de vertus, et on voyait paraître en cette jeune princesse plus de belles qualités qu'elle n'attendait de couronnes.... Philippe l'élève ainsi pour ses Etats; Dieu, qui nous aime, la destine à Louis" (212).

33. "Comment se conserve cette pureté dans ce lieu de tentations et parmi les illusions des grandeurs du monde, vous l'apprendrez de la Reine" (220).
34. "[C]e que je répète avec admiration, que les tendresses inexplicables de Marie-Thérèse tendaient toutes à lui inspirer la foi, la piété, la crainte de Dieu, un attachement inviolable pour le roi, des entrailles de miséricorde pour les malheureux, une immuable persévérance dans tous ses devoirs, et tout ce que louons dans la conduite de ce prince" (239).
35. "Toute cette gloire ne serait rien, si elle ne reposait pas sur un fond plus solide" (1283).
36. "C'est Dieu qui fait les guerriers et les conquérants" [God has made the warriors and the conquerors]; "Sans ce don inestimable de la piété, que serait-ce que le prince de Condé avec tout ce grand coeur et ce grand génie!" (370-371)
37. "Aussi avait-il pour maxime ...que dans les grands actions il faut uniquement songer à bien faire, et laisser venir la gloire après la vertu" (377).
38. "[T]out tendait au vrai et au grand. De là vient qu'il mettait sa gloire dans la service du roi et dans le bonheur de l'Etat:..." (377).
39. "[O] rois, confondez-vous dans votre grandeur; conquérants , ne vantez pas vos victoires" (390).
40. "Ce sont, ..., ces choses simples, gouverner sa famille, édifier ses domestiques, faire justice et miséricorde, accomplir le bien que Dieu veut, et souffrir les maux qu'il envoie, ce sont ces communes pratiques de la vie chrétienne que Jésus-Christ louera au dernier jour devant ses saints anges et devant son Père céleste" (396-397).
41. Davis, 19.
42. While Fénelon was at court, he became interested in Christian mysticism and, just as the king's mistress Madame de Maintenon had grown suspicious of the promoting of Quietism, he fell under the influence of Jeanne-Marie Bouvier de la Motte-Guyon. Mme Guyon was a spiritual writer, lay-woman mystic, and central figure in the controversy over Quietism, "a tendency within mystical theology that commends the soul's self-abandoning acceptance of whatever God sends ...and values silent contemplation above petitionary prayer" (660). Bossuet feared the potential of Quietism for moral indifference and passive emotionalism. Fénelon was shocked by his mentor's stance and appealed to wider opinion. Fénelon first approached Rome, then in his *Explication des maximes des saints* (1697), he attempted to refute point by point the disputed doctrines. Nevertheless, opinion at court turned against him. (Peter France, ed., *The New Oxford Companion to Literature in French* [Oxford: Clarendon Press, 1995], 307, 368, 660).
43. Davis, 66-67.
44. Davis, 64.
45. François de Salignac de la Mothe-Fénelon, *Les Aventures de Télémaque* (Paris: Garnier-Flammarion, 1968). All French citations are from this edition and will be noted with page numbers in the text.
46. "Ils [Hasaël et Mentor] continuèrent à parler de l'origine des dieux, des héros, des poètes, de l'âge de l'or, du déluge, des premières histoires du genre humain, du fleuve d'oubli où se plongent les âmes des morts, des peines éternelles préparées aux impies dans le gouffre noir du Tartare, et de cette heureuse paix dont jouissent les justes dans les Champs-Elysées, sans crainte de pouvoir la perdre" (135).
47. Patrick Riley, ed. & trans., *Telemachus, Son of Ulysses* (New York: Cambridge University Press, 1994), 56. The stories told by Mentor and Hasaël (a Syrian to whom Mentor had been sold as a slave) do not appear to be censored in the manner recommended by Plato in the *Republic*. In Book II, Socrates advocates telling the future guardians of the

city only those stories which are fine and beautiful, rejecting those which present bad images of gods and heroes (*Republic* 377c ff).

48. Volker Kapp, Télémaque *de Fénelon: la signification d'une oeuvre littéraire à la fin du siècle classique* (Tübingen: Gunter Narr, 1992). While *Telemachus* may very well have contributed to Fénelon's downfall, it was spectacularly successful. It was, after the Bible, the most read literary work in eighteenth-century France. It was praised by Rousseau; in *Emile*, Rousseau's pupil is given *Telemachus* upon reaching adulthood—"a striking concession from one who thought almost all literature morally suspect" (Riley xvii). *Telemachus* was translated into English in the year of its publication, and in 1776 it was rendered into English by no less than the novelist Tobias Smollett (Riley xvi-xvii).

49. Riley, xviii.

50. Riley, xxvii. In Homer's account, the goddess Athena went to Ithaca to prepare Telemachus to go on a journey in search of his father. Disguised as a sea-faring man, Athena appeared at Telemachus' door and advised him to try to find out something about his father's fate. Athena disguised herself as Mentor, whom Ulysses trusted the most of all Ithacans. Thus disguised, Athena promised to sail with Telemachus (Edith Hamilton, *Mythology* [New York: Mentor, 1940], 205-206).

51. François-Xavier Cuche, Télémaque *entre Père et mer* (Paris: Honoré Champion, 1995). In a letter from 1710, Fénelon himself indicates his objective in writing *Telemachus*:

> As for *Télémaque*, it is a fabulous narration in the form of an heroic poem like those of Homer and of Virgil, into which I have put the main instructions which are suitable for a young prince whose birth destines him to rule…. In these adventures I have put all the truths necessary to government, and all the faults that one can find in sovereign power. (Fénelon in a letter to Father LeTellier, in *Oeuvres*, 1835 ed., Vol. III, pp. 653-654; cited in Riley, xviii).

52. It may be tempting to label *Telemachus* as a piece of utopian literature. As Cuche points out, the principal functions of a utopian work are present in *Telemachus*: the normative function, which defines the rules of an ideal government; the critical function, which stimulates the political imagination by comparing models with reality; the experimental function, which allows political thought to begin to take shape, as a sort of *in vitro* verification of an idea; an esthetic function, which transforms society into something beautiful; and a mythical and religious function, which turns events toward their most pure essence, freeing them from accidents of history and from individual existence (150).

53. "Il peut tout sur les peuples; mais les lois peuvent tout sur lui. Il a une puissance absolue pour faire le bien, et les mains liées dès qu'il veut faire le mal" (142).

54. Cuche, 170. Bossuet had likewise pointed out that the king should be brought up respecting the law in order to avoid becoming a tyrant.

55. " 'Je ne connais qu'un seul moyen pour rendre votre people modeste dans sa dépense, c'est que vous lui en donniez vous-même l'exemple' …le sage Mentor lui fit remarquer que les lois mêmes, quoique renouvelées, seraient inutiles, si l'exemple du roi ne leur donnait une autorité qui ne pouvait venir d'ailleurs" (278).

56. "Il faut établir des écoles publiques, où l'on enseigne la crainte des dieux, l'amour de la patrie, le respect des lois, la préférence de l'honneur aux plaisirs et à la même" (287).

57. "La guerre est quelquefois nécessaire, il est vrai; mais c'est la honte du genre humain, qu'elle soit inévitable en certaines occasions. O rois, ne dites point qu'on doit la désirer pour acquérir de la gloire: la vraie gloire ne se trouve point hors de l'humanité" (258).

58. "[M]ais, de peur que toute la nation ne s'amollisse et ne tombe dans l'ignorance de la guerre, il faut envoyer dans les guerres étrangères la jeune noblesse. Ceux-là suffisent pour entretenir toute la nation dans une émulation de gloire, dans l'amour des armes, dans le mépris des fatigues et de la mort même, enfin dans l'expérience de l'art militaire" (269).

59. Davis, 109. Charles-Louis de Secondat, baron de la Brède et de Montesquieu, was born in 1689, into a noble family of the region of Bordeaux. His family had distinguished itself in the legal profession, particularly as members of the Bordeaux *parlement*.

60. "Il y avait en Arabie un petit peuple appelé Troglodyte, ...qui ...ressemblaient plus à des bêtes qu'à des hommes." Montesquieu, *Lettres persanes*, ed. Laurent Versini (Paris: GF-Flammarion, 1995), 53. All citations from the text are from this edition; references will be cited by page number only. I am particularly indebted to an article by Allessandro S. Crisafulli, "Montesquieu's Story of the Troglodytes: Its Background, Meaning, and Significance," *PMLA* LVIII, 2 (June 1943): 372-392, for a thorough explication of the Troglodyte letters.

61. Lester G. Crocker, *Nature and Culture: Ethical Thought in the French Enlightenment* (Baltimore: Johns Hopkins Press, 1963), 435.

62. Crocker, 490. Crocker continues his analysis by subdividing the second group into two subgroups: those who opposed enlightened despotism in favor of intermediary powers, and those who distrusted the intermediary powers and favored benevolent despots.

63. E.O. Wilson, "Back from Chaos," *The Atlantic Monthly* (March 1998). Online. Available. http://www.theatlantic.com/98mar/eowilson.htm.

64. Jean Bethke Elshtain, *Meditations on Modern Political Thought* (New York: Praeger, 1986), 38.

65. Jean Bethke Elshtain, *Democracy on Trial* (New York: BasicBooks, 1995), 9.

QUESTIONS FOR DISCUSSION

1. Bossuet drafted his instructions to a seventeenth-century ruler thought to be chosen by God. Are these instructions applicable for today's student in an egalitarian society where, theoretically, anyone can become a leader?

2. How might Bossuet's ideas about moral guidance be implemented in character education programs in today's schools?

3. Is Bossuet's leadership goal of cultivating a "happy people" an appropriate goal for today's political leaders?

4. To what attributes of character should the people of a democracy aspire? Is happiness an important attribute? What role should a leader play in assuring that people cultivate the right kinds of virtues?

5. Do democracies rely on encouraging a participatory public rather than a submissive one? If they do, how does this affect the leaders' responsibilities for the welfare of their public?

6. If we no longer consider our leaders to be "all-knowing" or "God-like," as leaders were seen in the past, will this necessarily have a negative impact on today's government and society?

ETHICS IN HISTORY: A FRENCH CONSCIENCE

Richard Francis Crane

ABSTRACT

The study of history often involves the study of ethical aspects of the human past. This essay reconstructs the memory of General Louis Eugène Faucher, a long-neglected hero of the Second World War. Faucher's outraged resistance to appeasement, capitulation, and collaboration led him to play a distinctive role in the tortured history of World War Two France. He stood virtually alone in denouncing the appeasement of Hitler and the abandonment of Czechoslovakia in September 1938. This ethical stance served as a prelude to playing a leadership role in the wartime French Resistance. Faucher's actions have consequently left an indelible mark of French courage as well as French shame on the memory of the Second World War, reminding us that doing the right thing in the face of evil is not always easy to do, but ultimately it is the only thing worth doing.

How does ethics make a difference in history? One might argue that ethics figures not only at the center of human actions comprising that thing we casually call history, but also enters into the sometimes difficult task of deciding what to remember (and how to remember it) as the "true" historical record. Consider the following statement from a French historian of the Second World War, which encapsulates both the exceptionality and awkward remembrance of those who joined the Resistance between 1940 and 1944[1]:

> The *résistant* is a fascinating and disturbing figure. He is not only a combatant in the world war, but he is also an actor in the war of Frenchmen against Frenchmen. His image is a double one, because he simultaneously embodies

the hero who saved the honor of France and living proof that the French, divided, did not immediately recognize themselves in him.[2]

Historians often construct and employ abstractions which, like the above passage, touch on ethical questions about both human behavior in the past and historical memory unto the present. After all, people not only make choices about what they do at a given moment in time, but people also decide in some manner or other how to remember and make sense of the historical past. But all this remains an abstraction until we employ the flesh and blood example of a French general and Resistance fighter, Louis Eugène Faucher.

APPEASING HITLER—THE PRICE OF PEACE?

Europe stood poised on the brink of war in September 1938, as Hitler vowed to unleash his Wehrmacht against Czechoslovakia, an East Central European state doubly offensive to the Nazi dictator both as the lone democracy in the region and as the home—or prison, as Hitler professed it—of over three million ethnic Germans. As in 1914, it seemed that the eruption of a violent conflict in one obscure part of Europe might well lead to the outbreak of a general, unstoppable war. At the height of the crisis Prime Minister Neville Chamberlain spoke to millions of terrified Britons huddled around their radios: "How horrible, fantastic, incredible it is that we should be digging trenches and trying on gas-masks here because of a quarrel in a far-away country between people of whom we know nothing."[3] Given the lingering trauma of the Great War, which cost the British nation three quarters of a million lives, and the French almost a million and a half dead, few people in these countries thought that any price could be counted as too high if it forestalled the coming of another horrific bloodletting.

The Czechoslovak Republic paid that price at the Munich Conference on 29 September 1938, when it lost the strategically vital Sudetenland, with its 3.25 million German-speaking inhabitants, to Hitler's Germany and accepted virtual satellite status *vis à vis* the Reich. Not that the Czechoslovaks had a say in this treaty—its signatories included the leaders of Germany, Italy, Britain, and Czechoslovakia's own ally France. But such quibbles took a back seat to the basic fact that the small sacrifice of Czechoslovak territorial integrity and national sovereignty had prevented another world war from breaking out. Hence the rapturous welcome accorded to Chamberlain when he returned to England and hence the near-universal acclaim for what has since become known as one of the most ethically-loaded words in the English language, appeasement.[4]

About a week before the Munich agreement took shape, at least one voice had been raised against the emerging policy of appeasement. On 23 September 1938, General Louis Eugène Faucher resigned his post as Chief of the French Military Mission in Prague and made ready to join the Czechoslovak Army in the field, where it was mobilizing to meet an expected German attack. Faucher's act served as a disavowal of the policies of his military and political superiors, policies which a week later would spawn the "Munich surrender." In the atmosphere of impending disaster and desperate hopes in France, Faucher's protest against the abandonment of Czechoslovakia received little public attention, while within the French high command it provoked a sharp letter of reprimand from Faucher's chief, General Maurice Gamelin, who wrote, "I level upon you the censure of the Chief of the General Staff, and urge you to continue to fulfill the duties of a French general." [5] Faucher replied that he had long considered one of those duties to be "that of always telling you the truth, without succumbing to the temptation to conceal it when I think it might be disagreeable to hear."[6] The truth, as Faucher saw it, fell on decidedly unreceptive ears in September 1938.

Today, when numerous historians have demonstrated the folly of appeasement as a policy intended to restrain Hitlerian aggression, the supposedly "quixotic" incident of Faucher's resignation rarely merits more than a sentence or two in even the most thorough studies of the coming of the Second World War. Yet the refusal of a senior French general to accept appeasement provides an illuminating contrast to the prevailing mood of escapism that characterized the French nation on the eve of the war. A "*Résistant* before the Resistance,"[7] Faucher stands out in a national climate of denial and debasement.[8] The Free French broadcaster Maurice Schumann would later write, "In truth, Louis Faucher was not the voice of our conscience in 1938. He was our conscience itself."[9]

Faucher's rejection of appeasement, far from being impulsive or sentimentally inspired, drew on several longer antecedents, including his role in France and Czechoslovakia's problematic interwar relations; his opposition to France's defensive strategic mentality as typified by the static fortifications of the Maginot Line; and finally, his own moral and intellectual development. Faucher's uncompromising stance in September 1938 had thus evolved over many years. And while the Munich crisis presented him with a difficult choice between the dictates of moral conscience and the constraints of military discipline, his resignation did not mark the end of his career; instead, it signified the beginning of his own journey toward what would eventually be called the Resistance.

THE MILTARY MISSION IN PRAGUE, 1919-38

Faucher's involvement in Franco-Czechoslovak relations began in the wake of the Great War when he arrived in Prague in February 1919 as one of forty-five volunteer officers comprising the French Military Mission to newly independent Czechoslovakia. The advisory group's mission went beyond altruism, for strengthening the infant republic promised to enhance French aims of containing Germany and stemming the Bolshevik tide in the east. But even as Mission Chief General Maurice Pellé[10] and his officers assumed command of Czechoslovakia's forces after a Hungarian communist invasion in summer 1919, the Czechoslovaks resisted the excesses of French influence. When French forces occupied the German industrial heartland known as the Ruhr in January 1923, the French government and general staff counted on their eastern allies to support them against Germany. But the feuding Poles and Czechoslovaks emphasized their ongoing territorial squabbling instead of backing France in the contest over reparations, the financial penalties Germany owed the victorious Allies from World War I.

Then the independent diplomacy of Czechoslovak Foreign Minister Edvard Benes restricted the January 1924 Franco-Czechoslovak Treaty to a vague political accord lacking the binding military clauses Paris craved at that time. The Prague authorities also welcomed the October 1925 Locarno Pact, an agreement that apparently reconciled Czechoslovakia's key ally France with the Czechoslovaks' number-one trading partner, Germany. Czechoslovakia's subsequent warmer relations with Germans inside and outside its borders also demanded that French officers cease to command its troops. In January 1926 the Mission's second chief, General Eugène Mittelhausser, returned home as the Mission resumed a strictly advisory role under Brigadier General Louis Eugène Faucher.[11]

As the institution of the Mission receded in importance, the influence and authority of its chief increased. Faucher worked alongside new Chief of Staff General Jan Syrovy in refining the Czechoslovak Army and joined in the deliberations of the five-man National Defense Council convened weekly at the presidential palace. Given the lack of explicit formal ties between France and Czechoslovakia, and the fact that France posted five different ministers in Prague in the thirteen years between the signing of the Locarno and Munich treaties, Faucher's close long-term standing amongst the Czechoslovaks—who came to call him "our General Faucher"[12]—necessarily entailed a degree of political significance.

At the same time, Faucher periodically suggested to his superiors in Paris that the Mission be dissolved, citing the conclusion of its purely military functions in Czechoslovakia. In 1929-30 career considerations also demanded that he assume a required field command in France before receiving another general's star. Nevertheless, the Czechoslovak and French foreign ministries simultaneously intervened, since neither his own nor the Czechoslovak government wanted him to leave his post. Hence, the apparently indispensable Faucher remained in Prague, receiving two more stars in the next four years. And between 1936 and 1938 the two governments blocked the sexagenarian general's mandatory retirement from the ranks; Faucher's irreplaceability demanded an exception to regulations to which General Gamelin fully agreed. The retention of Faucher in his post in Prague helped mask the shortcomings in Franco-Czechoslovak relations and also increased the depth of the Mission Chief's long-developing dual allegiance, two factors behind Faucher's eventual response to the Munich crisis.[13]

Faucher also resisted the development of French military strategy in the 1930s. Gamelin's assumption of the top army post of inspector general in January 1935 did not in any way alter France's inward-looking strategic doctrine of *défense intégrale*, except that it prompted a modification of Gamelin's predecessor General Maxime Weygand's thesis that only a militarily strong France could survive another war of attrition. The new commander, avoiding budgetary battles with the politicians, asserted that real security lay not in the mere stockpiling of arms but in pursuing and cultivating alliances. France could only hold its own in a war with a larger, stronger Germany if it could be assured of the strength of a coalition and the solace of multiple alternate battlefields. Frequent ministerial changes, the growing bitter rift between Left and Right, and widespread antipathy toward the parliamentary regime led embattled and distracted governmental leaders to increase their reliance on seasoned military experts in the formulation of foreign policy. Given this relative decline of civilian authority in the 1930s, political leaders tended to agree to postpone indefinitely French entry into any battle not directly forced upon the country.[14]

Even if war proved unavoidable, France would keep its forces on the defensive behind the Maginot fortifications until the time seemed right to render the decision against a Germany bled white by multi-front warfare and starved by blockade. The "blood of others,"[15] that is, those lucky enough to have been France's allies at the time, would buy time in what came to be called *la guerre de longue durée*, a war of long duration like the 1914-18 conflict. As the French high command coolly forecast the "initial pulverization"[16] of

France's ally Czechoslovakia, Faucher asserted that French passivity promised to undermine the very alliances upon which French strategy rested. Unable to move beyond his narrowly constructed strategic vision, Gamelin wrongly saw an unopposed Rhineland reoccupation by the German Army as essential to binding together a mutually-alarmed anti-German coalition. But Faucher correctly judged Hitler's 7 March 1936 move as the opening salvo of the Second World War, another indication of French abdication in the face of the Reich.[17]

Faucher also argued against discounting the military value of the Soviet Union, even as the dominant members of the French high command railed against Stalinist perfidy and Moscow's pernicious control of the French Communist Party. Deputy Chief of Staff General Victor Schweisguth suspected the worst from reports of Czechoslovak-Soviet military and political contacts and ordered Faucher to get to the bottom of the rumors. The Mission Chief countered by insisting that one could hardly blame the Czechoslovaks for thinking that lukewarm French support hardly sufficed now that the Reich was on the march. France's simultaneously self-serving and self-defeating military policies found themselves influenced by the high command's ideological predilections to hold onto the illusion of an alliance with fascist Italy even as Mussolini became an ever closer ally of Hitler. And even with Italy drifting into the Hitlerian camp, most French generals still rejected out of hand any cooperation with the vastly more powerful Soviets, deemed dangerous and unpredictable because of their communism. As an early partisan of a "grand alliance" against Hitler, Faucher thought it nonsensical to neglect any potential partner against German aggression. A consequent sense of frustration verging on outrage fueled Faucher's growing criticism of his superiors.[18]

Faucher's own life history also inspired his resistance to appeasement. Born on 8 October 1874 to a peasant family in the western *département* of Deux-Sèvres, he prepared to follow his father into woodworking until he won a government-sponsored scholarship competition. The *boursier* (government scholarship recipient) owed his good fortune to the young Third Republic, and his attachment to republican values would later lead his fellow junior officers to nickname him "the Democrat." Faucher's ensuing dedication to his studies, particularly mathematics, opened the doors of the *Ecole polytechnique*, where he trained to become an army engineer. Commissioned a second lieutenant in October 1896, Faucher led an engineer battalion before joining Marshal Philippe Pétain's staff at the Battle of Verdun, the fiercest of the First World War. Emerging alive in 1918 as a lieutenant colonel, he embarked for Prague.[19]

Faucher lived and worked in the Czechoslovak capital for nearly twenty years, where he soon mastered Czech and immersed himself in every aspect of the country's ongoing life and historical legacy of struggle. A Protestant, Faucher identified with a state that inherited its motto, "Truth Prevails," from the fifteenth-century Hussite movement, a movement of religious protest. And one historian has observed that the Mission Chief's "deep Protestant rigor"[20] earned the respect and trust of his Czechoslovak counterparts.

If Faucher's political allegiance defies precise identification, it is because he embraced democracy more as a transcendent moral creed than as a sectarian attachment to party. Accordingly, the pan-humanist President-Liberator Tomas Masaryk, "a seeker of truth," stood as perhaps the greatest influence on him. He considered himself "a student of Masaryk,"[21] and the death of the founding father of Czechoslovakia in September 1937 shook both Faucher and the Czechoslovak population at large. At the same time, the bitter polarization of French democracy, with its resultant foreign-policy impotence, continued. As Czechoslovakia faced the growing Nazi threat, Faucher's earlier questioning of French capabilities and intentions gave way to moral outrage.

THE PATH TO RESISTANCE, 1938-45

For these reasons, Faucher's resignation in the midst of the Munich crisis should be seen in the context of its longer origins, particularly if one is to grasp fully its ethical dimensions. Moreover, Faucher's subsequent career points to his response to Munich as his first step toward the Resistance. When France joined Great Britain in allowing Czechoslovakia to be forced into the German orbit, both the European balance of power and the nature of the Czechoslovak state were bound to change. The rump state of Czecho-Slovakia now became an authoritarian puppet of the Third Reich. In October Faucher tried to intercede with the Czecho-Slovak government to prevent anti-Nazi refugees from the Sudetenland (many of them Jews) from being turned over to the Gestapo. But as General Jan Syrovy, now premier, coldly informed Faucher: "we have been willing to fight on the side of the angels, now we shall hunt with the wolves."[22]

This emotionally wrenching turn of events only galvanized the former Mission Chief's resentment toward compromise with Hitler. In her novel *A Stricken Field*, Martha Gellhorn depicted the General Faucher she knew in Prague (his name fictionalized as "General Labonne") as a man who had prepared himself for the possibility of ending up in a Nazi concentration camp "as if the idea delighted him." But this should perhaps be seen more as a literary flourish than a penetrating observation of Faucher's psyche. More realistically, Faucher eagerly anticipated the challenge of resistance, while he fully realized the risks involved. After the celebrated American war reporter left Prague she continued to correspond with the General, whom she considered "far the best and cleanest man anywhere."[23]

Faucher's last unhappy weeks in Prague concluded with his December departure, an event applauded in the Nazi German press as the true end of the "Benes era" (Benes himself had resigned and left the country soon after Munich). Recent personal and professional tragedy notwithstanding, Faucher treated his retirement as a beginning, immediately setting to work against the continued illusions and dangers of appeasement. Shortly before Christmas, he sat down to an interview with journalist Henri de Kerillis, a conservative deputy who alone had voted against ratifying the Munich treaty. Faucher indicted the French defeatism behind Munich and accused some of the journalists of the far Right of taking many of their ideas, and much of their pay, from Berlin.[24] Faucher then spoke at London's Royal Institute of International Affairs on 23 February 1939. The former French general identified himself as "one of those who wish to establish less vacillating standards of moral values in international politics."[25]

His message, that Czechoslovakia's dangers were all Europe's and that the mutilated republic should be preserved from final destruction, seems all the more poignant and pertinent for its sad timing. On 16 March, after a lightning invasion that met no resistance, Hitler and his army stood in Prague, the swastika banner flying over the presidential palace in what had been East Central Europe's last surviving democracy. After Hitler discarded the mask of peaceful seeker of national justice he had worn to the Munich Conference, even the arch-appeaser Neville Chamberlain could hardly deny the inevitability of war. On 3 September 1939 France and Great Britain declared war upon Germany after the latter's attack on Poland. Soviet Russia, previously shut out of western security planning,[26] in spite of Faucher's remonstrances, remained neutral as Europe plunged into another world war.

As French and British forces awaited the Nazi onslaught in the West (their defensive doctrines and belated rearmament disposed them to do little else), Faucher found himself summoned from retirement to help form a Czechoslovak army in France. As chief of a new French Military Mission, he drew on his long experience and rapport with his Czechoslovak comrades. An April 1940 article in the *Revue des Deux Mondes* described Faucher's position amongst the volunteers as follows: "Officers and soldiers alike consider him the father of their army, and have absolute faith in him."[27] Their confidence proved well-founded when, in the chaos of the June 1940 defeat, Faucher ignored the new Pétain government's orders to dissolve the Mission, insisting on remaining at his post until all Czechoslovak soldiers, whom the Germans promised to shoot as traitors, embarked for England and safety. One Czechoslovak soldier recalled seeing "that legendary figure, briskly marching among us, trying to see and talk to as many of our soldiers and officers as possible," insisting that without Faucher's involvement it would have been "doubtful whether we would have found our way from the middle and muddle of the French debacle."[28] After the Armistice Faucher joined thousands of officers in retirement, but he also numbered among the smaller group that comprised the military resistance organization, *L'Armée secrète*. As the General's son describes it, Faucher's disgust at the antisemitism and collaborationism of many of his countrymen led him to pursue resistance activities "to an almost suicidal degree."[29]

Faucher commanded the Secret Army in his native Deux-Sèvres,[30] where under the codename "Thomas" he also coordinated the resistance activities of the left-of-center *Libération* and the conservative *Organisation Civile et Militaire*. Heavy losses in the "shadow war" were exacerbated by confessions under German torture, and on 29 January 1944 Faucher found himself betrayed and captured. The Gestapo entered his home shortly after a colleague gave him a list of regional resistance contacts. Luckily his captors consented to a change of footwear, after which the crumpled paper containing the names of numerous other resisters remained behind in his slippers. Though he thereby saved several lives, Faucher, then in his seventieth year, despaired of his own. Imprisoned in Poitiers, then deported to Godesberg (the site of one of Hitler and Chamberlain's pre-Munich meetings), and finally brought to the Tyrol, the aged prisoner had only Caesar's *Gallic Wars* and the Bible for intellectual and spiritual nourishment. During this time of fear and hardship he underwent what he subsequently identified as his true conversion experience; doubtless his faith helped him survive until American troops liberated him at the end of the war.[31]

General Charles de Gaulle wrote the repatriated Faucher on 1 August 1945 in words that evoked their shared devotion to their country and its ideals. "You and I," de Gaulle pronounced, "are fated to make sure that France never again debases herself, never again lets fall her glory."[32] These are ringing words to be sure, but Faucher had embraced this mission and burned his bridges long before de Gaulle and others took up the challenge after the fall of France in 1940. By September 1938, this French general asserted that war had already begun, even as the vast majority of his compatriots hoped and believed that a fight with Hitler could still be averted. A *"Résistant* before the Resistance," Louis Eugène Faucher was perhaps the first to face a choice that many French men and women of conscience would eventually have to make. Faucher personifies the conclusion that resistance to appeasement in 1938 anticipated resistance to capitulation and collaboration after 1940.

WHY FAUCHER?

William Butler Yeats wrote the following poetic words during the interwar period which have since come to encapsulate the ethical-political failures of democratic societies threatened by ruthless dictatorships: "The best lack all conviction, while the worst are full of passionate intensity."[33] But Yeats had never met General Faucher, a meeting which had it happened might well have inspired the poet to add a qualifying line or two to his very evocative work. After all, the example of Faucher offers us a retrospective "way out" of the ethical dilemmas of that "decade of swine"[34] known as the Thirties, and one which might at first glance seem deceptively simple: courage in the face of evil.

Why is the case of Faucher important ethically and historically? It is because his rejection of appeasement has left an indelible mark of French courage as well as French shame on the memory of the Second World War, a conflict central to the history of the twentieth century. In other words, Faucher can be seen as a bright spot within a dark memory, for he went against the currents of history around him, currents he could see more clearly than most of his contemporaries. Accordingly we are reminded that dealing with ethical questions involves a kind of transcendence. In transcending narrow self-interest, we may achieve a clarity of vision in perceiving the greater good. Yet even once we see, reacting courageously is much more easily said than done.

In terms of finding the strength to take the ultimate life-and-death ethical stance as a member of the French Resistance, Faucher's courage was not found wanting. His lesson to his contemporaries still resonates as a lesson to us today. Doing the right thing is not always easy, but in the final analysis it is the only thing worth doing. In Plato's *Republic,* Socrates tells us that "courage is a kind of preservation."[35] With all that the world lost in the Second World War, we should count ourselves lucky that some few individuals from the beginning sought to preserve the democratic and humanitarian ideals really worth fighting for; and they did so until the majority belatedly shared in this realization. With that remembrance, General Faucher remains before us not simply as an object lesson of ethics in history, but also as a teacher.

NOTES

1. Direct quotations in this paper have been translated as needed from the original French by the author. More extensive historiographical citations can be found in Richard Francis Crane, *A French Conscience in Prague: Louis Eugène Faucher and the Abandonment of Czechoslovakia*. (Boulder: East European Monographs, 1996).
2. Robert Frank, "La Mémoire empoisonnée," in Jean-Pierre Azéma and François Bédarida, eds., *La France des Années Noires. Tome 2. De l'Occupation à la Libération* (Paris: Seuil, 1993), 489.
3. Chamberlain radio address of 27 September 1938 reprinted in *Peace or Appeasement? Hitler, Chamberlain, and the Munich Crisis*, ed. Francis L. Lowenheim (Boston: Houghton Mifflin, 1965), 55.
4. The following still serves as a good, though exhaustive, introduction: Telford Taylor, *Munich: The Price of Peace* (Garden City, NY: Doubleday, 1979).
5. Service Historique de l'Armée de Terre Française, Vincennes (henceforth SHA), 7N3115, Telegram from Gamelin to Faucher, 25 September 1938.
6. *Documents Diplomatiques Français, 1932-1939, 2ième Série, Tome XII* (Paris, 1963), Document 49, Letter from Faucher to Gamelin, 6 October 1938.
7 Author's interview with Madame Marie de Lacroix-Rist, daughter of French Minister in Prague M. Victor de Lacroix (1935-1939), Paris, August 1991. The author thanks the late Madame de Lacroix-Rist for the evocative phrase "un résistant avant la Résistance."
8. Yvon Lacaze has published two authoritative studies on France and Munich: *L'opinion publique française et la crise de Munich* (Berne: Peter Lang, 1991); and *La France et Munich: Etude d'un processus décisionnel en matière de relations internationales*. (Berne: Peter Lang, 1992). The latter book can be found in English translation as well: *France and Munich: A Study of Decision Making in International Affairs* (Boulder: East European Monographs, 1995).
9. Maurice Schumann, "Louis Faucher devant notre conscience et devant l'histoire," in E.V. Faucher, ed., *Louis Eugène Faucher* (privately published, 1967), 7.
10. The author thanks Madame Mariska Sandiford-Pellé for kindly sending the author the gift of an inscribed copy of a long out-of-print biography of her father: Lieutenant-Colonel de Thomasson, *Le Général Pellé* (Paris: Gauthier-Villars, 1933).
11. SHA 7N3097, Faucher report, "La Mission Militaire Française auprès de la République Tchécoslovaque (1919-1938): Rapport de fin de Mission," 15 December 1938. See also Philippe Hauser, *De la Gloire à la Désillusion: Les rélations politiques et militaires franco-tchécoslovaques du Traité de Versailles à la crise de Munich (1919-1938)* (Paris: Vécu Contemporain, 1996). The author thanks M. Hauser for sending him a copy of this book.
12. Piotr Wandycz, *The Twilight of French Eastern Alliances, 1926-1936* (Princeton: Princeton University Press, 1988), 462.
13. Crane, *A French Conscience in Prague*, 52-53, 89-90.

12. Piotr Wandycz, *The Twilight of French Eastern Alliances, 1926-1936* (Princeton: Princeton University Press, 1988), 462.
13. Crane, *A French Conscience in Prague*, 52-53, 89-90.
14. Nicole Jordan, "The Cut Price War on the Peripheries: The French General Staff, the Rhineland, and Czechoslovakia," in *Paths To War: New Essays on the Origins of the Second World War*, edited by Robert Boyce and Esmonde M. Robertson (New York: St. Martin's, 1989), 128-166.
15. See Nicole Jordan, *The Popular Front and Central Europe: The Dilemmas of French Impotence, 1918-1940* (New York: Cambridge University Press, 1992). Further impressions of Gamelin as a strategist can be gleaned from Martin Alexander, *The Republic in Danger: General Maurice Gamelin and the Politics of French Defence* (New York: Cambridge University Press, 1993).
16. SHA 2N20, "Etude sur l'établissement de plans de défense nationale dans les différentes hypothèses de conflit."
17. Crane, *A French Conscience in Prague*, 77-78.
18. Ibid., 68-93.
19. Ibid., 12-15.
20. Antoine Mares, "La faillite des rélations franco-tchécoslovaques: la mission militaire française à Prague (1926-1938), *Revue d'Histoire de la Deuxième Guerre Mondiale* 111 (1978), 57.
21. Both quotes excerpted from a radio address reprinted as "Le général Faucher parle aux Tchèques et aux Slovaques," *L'Amitié Franco-Tchécoslovaque* 14.2 (April-June 1963).
22. Sir John Wheeler-Bennett, *Knaves, Fools, and Heroes* (London: Macmillan, 1974), 144.
23. Martha Gellhorn, *A Stricken Field* (New York: Virago, 1986), 198, 308. The author thanks the late Ms. Gellhorn for her additional insights so kindly given over five years of correspondence.
24. Crane, *A French Conscience in Prague*, 155.
25. General Faucher, "Some Recollections of Czecho-Slovakia," *International Affairs* XVIII (May-June 1939), 343-360.
26. See Michael Jabara Carley, "End of the 'Low, Dishonest Decade': Failure of the Anglo-Franco-Soviet Alliance in 1939," *Europe-Asia Studies*, 45,5 (1993), 303-341.
27. Robert Vaucher, "L'Armée tchécoslovaque de France," *Revue des Deux Mondes*, 1 April 1940, 551-556.
28. Letter, General M.F. Kaspar to author, 11 November 1994. He goes on to write: "Again, the same distinct small figure wearing the horizon-bleu and the képi was the last object we saw on the quay of Sète as our Egyptian cargo ship under the British flag was leaving for Gibraltar, carrying an improbable number of over 3000 Czechoslovak troops." Other Czechoslovak World War Two veterans have expressed to this author similar appreciative feelings about Faucher and the "true France" he represented.
29. Author's interview with Professor Eugène Vaçlav Faucher, St. Maixent, July 1995. The author is grateful to the Faucher family both for their hospitality and for allowing him to see the previously closed Faucher private papers.
30. On the subject of resistance movements in Deux-Sèvres, see Michel Chaumet and Jean-Marie Pouplain, *La Résistance en Deux-Sèvres, 1940-1944* (Parthenay: Geste Editions, 1994).
31. Crane, *A French Conscience in Prague*, 157-158.
32. SHA 1K288, Letter from de Gaulle to Faucher, 1 August 1945.

33. "The Second Coming," in *Selected Poems and Two Plays of William Butler Yeats*, edited by M.L. Rosenthal (New York: Collier, 1962), 91.
34. Igor Lukes, *Czechoslovakia between Stalin and Hitler: The Diplomacy of Edvard Benes in the 1930s* (New York: Oxford University Press, 1996), 263.
35. Plato, *Republic*, trans. G.M.A. Grube, rev. C.D.C. Reeve (Indianapolis: Hackett, 1992), 104.

QUESTIONS FOR DISCUSSION

1. What gave Louis Eugène Faucher the courage to break the chain of command? Does a good military man always follow orders?

2. Faucher had a longstanding relationship with Czechoslovakia. Does one require personal involvement with a person, group, or nation in order to advocate for justice or take courageous stands?

3. What does it mean for nations to cultivate relationships and develop alliances, but then refuse to engage in military battles that might result from these engagements?

4. How did Faucher's early life experiences prepare him for the ethical challenges that lay ahead of him during the 1938-45 period?

5. What might the transcendent democratic ideas be that shaped Faucher's moral creed?

6. What heroic attributes did Faucher possess? Who are our heroes? Why? What are their qualities?

7. The Second World War is sometimes called the "Good War." Does the case of Faucher support this assessment?

ANCIENT WISDOM FOR EDUCATORS AND PARENTS: PROVERBIAL WISDOM FROM SOCRATES, THE OLD TESTAMENT, AND CONFUCIUS

John Hemphill

ABSTRACT

The purposes of this paper are (1) to compare the ethical themes found in the teachings of Socrates, Confucius and the biblical book of Proverbs, and (2) to show the existence of a universal, ethical foundation. The paper begins with a review of the historical role that schooling has played in the development of character, then proceeds to a discussion of each of the three sources of ancient wisdom. The review of each source points out the common ethical themes and provides information about the connection between wisdom and the development of character within each of the three cultures. The paper ends with some thoughts about how ancient wisdom could be used in today's public schools.

As the century closes on an American school system burdened by a perception that discipline and order are missing from the typical school, the characters of both our children and their schools are called into question. To help cope with the potential for disrespectful and violent students, many schools are implementing some form of character education, an intentional effort to develop ethical behaviors and habits. Is character development within the realm of responsibility for public schools? Many Americans believe it is. However, many educators and parents are concerned about whether or not there is a common ethical ground that provides a foundation for character education in the public school. Any formal character education curriculum would need to reflect the ethical values of the significant ethnic groups and cultures served by public schools. The purpose of this paper is to examine three different ancient sources of wisdom to see if there is, among the three sources, evidence of a universal, ethical foundation.

Since an effort will be made to connect ancient wisdom to modern schooling, a brief review is provided of the historical role schools have played in the development of character. The history of American education has, until recently, been consistent about character education. Prior to the middle of the twentieth century, it would have seemed irrational to speak of character education as something to add to the curriculum. The vast majority of parents and teachers have always assumed character development was an element and product of schooling. Public schooling in America dates back to 1642, when the Massachusetts Bay Colony passed a law requiring parents to educate their children.[1] The purpose of the early schools, particularly in New England, was to teach children to read so they could understand the Bible. Even when public schooling became more commonly available in the nineteenth century and began to serve economic and political purposes, religious and moralistic lessons and literature were still common in the curriculum. The emphasis on morality can easily be found in the best selling textbook of the nineteenth century, *The McGuffey Readers*, which sold 122 million copies from 1836 to 1922.[2] These readers included Bible stories, the Lord's Prayer, and many didactic pieces that emphasized the moral themes of mercy, charity, industriousness, courage and thrift.[3]

Prior to the emergence of a comprehensive American school system, formal education was a function of religious institutions like the church or synagogue. Even after an inclusive and secular public school system developed in the United States, public school teachers were expected to maintain order and provide moral guidance. They were empowered to provide discipline and to instill respect. Teachers could use various means to achieve that end, including paddle, proverb and prayer.

Although most educators, today, do not believe public school should include religion in the curriculum or should use corporal punishment, most of us would agree that order and discipline are harder to achieve today than 30 years ago. We see many reasons for this decline, including social problems like divorce, poverty, drugs, television viewing, and the disintegration of community life.

No matter what one believes about the state of our public schools, its history or its potential, the possibility of including character education in the curriculum should be considered. This article presents a perspective on character education from ancient sages, with the goal of offering some clarity and guidance to what parents and educators should expect of public schools in the twenty-first century.

Institutionalized education, better called *schooling*, precedes the Christian era. It has its primary origins in the Greek gymnasium (a school for boys) and academy (a university).[4] The first part of this paper is an examination of the relationship between schooling and character formation in the Hellenic world of Socrates. The second section presents a discussion of the book of Proverbs as a text used for the instruction of the young in the ancient Hebraic culture. The third part presents some of the teachings of Confucius that pertain to the relationship between instruction and character formation.[5] The life of Confucius (551-479 B.C.E) in ancient China is roughly contemporaneous with that of Socrates (470?-399 B.C.E.) and the anonymous compiler(s) of the book of Proverbs (722-609 B.C.E). Though Confucius had no awareness of Socrates or the Hebraic scribes who compiled Proverbs, they lived at a similar point in the development of civilization: near the beginning of the historical record of their cultures. More importantly, for purposes related to this paper, the primary objection to character education is that we are so culturally diverse that we cannot agree on the "what" and the "how-to" of character education. Since we tend to think of eastern and western cultures as quite different, the section of this paper on the teachings of Confucius leads us to the conclusions and the thesis of this paper: If we examine the virtues taught by our cultural ancestors, we find the common ground of virtue and find that character development has always been an important educational goal.

SOCRATES AND GREEK SCHOOLING

Socrates left no written documents. We know him through Plato's Socratic dialogues and through the writings of other Greek philosophers. In Plato's *Republic* (ca. 380 B.C.E.),[6] Socrates spoke about the role of education. At many points in the dialogue with his pupils and friends, he made the case for education as essential to the health of the state.

In the ideal world of Socrates, the state would be ruled by a philosopher-king who was compelled to rule because of his wisdom and love of his state. The philosopher-king would be aided by a ruling class of well-educated "guardians."[7] Together, the philosopher-king and the guardians would be responsible for maintaining the order and integrity of education. Socrates insisted they be diligent in their responsibility for schooling and carefully consider the addition of any new content or methodology.

> Those in charge must cling to education and see that it isn't corrupted without their noticing it. Above all they must guard as carefully as they can against any innovation in music and poetry or in physical training that is counter to the established order. (424b)

Music, poetry, songs, stories, and physical training were the standard subjects of the curriculum. In *The Republic*, Socrates described the nature of the curriculum. At the beginning of Book III he quoted numerous lines from Homer's *Odyssey,* lines he believed should be omitted for young students, because the violence would cause them to grow up fearful or because the characters in the epic poem speak too irreverently about the gods. In today's world, Socrates would be a forceful advocate for the V-chips as a device to help parents restrict the television programming viewed by their children.

In describing the ideal *Republic*, Socrates empowered the state with pervasive control over individual lives. He appeared to make a distinction between education and upbringing:

> Good education and upbringing, when they are preserved, produce good natures. (424a)

The concepts are obviously related. It could be inferred that *upbringing* is the less formal of the two, that education refers to a more institutionalized process delivered by the gymnasium.

Socrates believed parents could not be trusted to provide the appropriate nurturing and training of children. Failure to exercise control over the rearing of children would put the order of society at risk:

> Those with the best natures become outstandingly bad when they receive a bad upbringing. (491e)

His solution to the problem of ineffective parenting was to make the state responsible for the rearing of children, rather than their biological parents.[8] As such an idea strikes us, today, as unrealistic, so it did to Socrates' pupils. But remember his pedagogy, his teaching strategy. As a teacher, he was a provocateur. He began with difficult questions and problems. He listened to his students' answers and solutions and challenged them to justify and to account for their contradictions. When his students challenged him, then the dialogue was on and true education was unfolding.

For Socrates, education was necessary for the state to become a just place and for an individual to achieve a happy and virtuous life. He believed everyone had the capacity to learn:

> The power to learn is present in everyone's soul. (518c)

However, he did not believe human nature was innately good. Education was necessary for people to gain self-control and to develop awareness of the good:

> Education takes for granted that sight is there but that it isn't turned in the right way or looking where it ought to look, and it tries to redirect it appropriately. (518d)

Socrates expressed ideas about the content and method of the curriculum that would be regarded as quite modern. For children, learning must be made enjoyable:

> Don't use force to train the children in these subjects; use play instead. That way you will see better what each of them is naturally suited for. (536e)

> No free person should learn anything like a slave. Forced bodily labor does no harm to the body, but nothing taught by force stays in the soul. (536e)

As children grow older, the subjects they learn should shift from music, poetry and physical training to mathematics:

> How sophisticated is the subject of calculation and how many ways it is useful for our purposes, provided that one practices it for the sake of knowing rather than trading. (525d)

As education progresses to more rigorous study, learning becomes challenging and not everyone is able to meet the challenge:

> People's souls give up more easily in hard study than in physical training, since the pain—being peculiar to them and not shared with their body—is more their own. (535b)

At the highest level, learning becomes a task of integrating knowledge and applying it toward a better, more virtuous life:

> The subjects they learned in no particular order as children they must now bring together to form a unified vision of their kinship both with one another and with the nature of that which is. (537c)

Finally, the degree to which Socrates linked education and the development of character cannot be overstated. Schooling was for the purpose of training the citizens of the state and for making philosophers of the guardians and rulers. For Socrates, philosophy was mainly an examination of the "good," which he expressed as the commonly recognized virtues of justice, courage, moderation, friendship and wisdom. To let Socrates speak for himself on these matters, the following represents proverbial wisdom Plato attributes to Socrates:[9]

> Injustice...causes civil war, hatred, and fighting among themselves, while *justice* brings friendship and a sense of common purpose. (351d)
> The most *courageous* and most rational soul is least disturbed or altered by any outside affection. (381a)
>
> *Moderation* is surely a kind of order, the mastery of certain kinds of pleasures and desires. (429e)
>
> *Friends* possess everything in common. (424a)
>
> Isn't it also generally true of *just people* that, towards the end of each course of action, association, or life, they enjoy a good reputation and collect the prizes from other human beings? (613c)

If Socrates were alive today, he would, in some respects, make a good superintendent of education, except for his theoretical problem with parents and his real problem with politicians. Though Socrates is not around to lead our school systems, he provides us with a model of an educator and citizen. Teachers today can use his pedagogy, which we know as Socratic dialogue. His ethical principles can be linked to biblical and Confucian wisdom. When the similarities among these ancient sources are recognized, we find the center for a character education curriculum.

CHARACTER EDUCATION FROM
THE COURT OF KING SOLOMON

The book of Proverbs dates back to Solomon's reign, about 950 B.C.E.;[10] but its existence as a written document can only be traced by biblical scholars to the reign of Hezekiah, somewhere between 722 and 609 B.C.E.[11] The first verse attributes the book's wisdom to King Solomon, "The proverbs of Solomon, son of David, king of Israel" (Prov. 1:1). The next three verses state the purpose of the collected wisdom:[12]

> For learning about wisdom and instruction, for understanding words of insight, for gaining instruction in wise dealing, righteousness, justice and equity; to teach shrewdness to the simple, knowledge and prudence to the young. (1:2-4)

Proverbs is not a single collection of proverbs but is a compilation of proverbs from at least four different sources, two different collections attributed to Solomon, then collections attributed to Agur and to King Lemuel's mother. Some segments of the book are not proverbs but are longer passages that serve as introductions to sets of proverbs, elaborations on moral principles, or—in one case—a story, complete with character, setting, and conflict. There appear to be more than four collections within the text because there are considerably more than four introductory passages.

Different sections of Proverbs have different moral emphases. Some passages focus on the nature of justice and the practical operation of a court system; some emphasize the connection between reverence for the LORD and living a virtuous life; some contain multiple warnings about sexual promiscuity, adultery, and the hazards of strong drink; some are concerned with foolishness and the various ways a young person can stray from a righteous life. Regardless of the varying themes and styles of the different collections, the book stands as a collection of wisdom and instruction directed primarily toward the young, but useful also for a person of any age seeking advice and direction. It is a text for learning and teaching, whether the teacher is a parent or an adult leader of the community.

We can only speculate about what kind of schooling might have existed in ancient Israel. The development of the large body of wisdom literature that exists in various books of the Old Testament would have required some institution to develop and preserve knowledge. The agents of such an institution existed in the Israelite monarchy. The administration of the monarchy required advisers, secretaries, planners and apparently historians and collectors.[13] But who were the teachers of the young? How and when were boys and girls instructed? According to Williams the Hebrew term for school, *beit ha-midrash* (literally, "house of study") does not occur in biblical literature and does not appear in print until about 180 B.C.E.[14] Prior to the appearance of a word for school, we can only guess that any education of the young that occurred outside the family might have taken place in, as Williams says, "an informal public space, such as a quiet corner of the market-place or a room at the Temple or at the home of a community leader."[15] The Temple was a place of learning and study primarily for adults, but a story from the New Testament tells us that Jesus, as a young boy, was permitted to sit in the Temple and learn from the rabbis.[16]

Though we have no way of knowing for sure what form of school might have existed in Jewish culture before the second century B.C.E., the words in Proverbs emphasize the family as a primary source of education of the young. Time and again the book exhorts the young to pay attention to the instruction of their parents:

> Hear, my child, your father's instruction, and do not reject your mother's teaching; for they are a fair garland for your head, and pendants for your neck (1: 8-9).

Many verses begin with the form of address, "My son, ..."

> My son, if you accept my words and store up my commands within you, turning your ear to wisdom and applying your heart to understanding .... (2:1-2)

The fact that the terms father and son occur more frequently than mother or daughter reflects the gender roles and relationships of that time. From the perspective of this Old Testament book, boys were in more need of instruction and woman was the source of wisdom. The usual noun of address is masculine (e.g., "my son" above) but wisdom itself is always personified as female.

> Wisdom has built her house, she has hewn her seven pillars. She has slaughtered her animals, she has mixed her wine, she has also set her table. She has sent out her servant-girls, she calls from the highest places in the town, "You that are simple, turn in here!" (9:1-4)

Though masculine nouns and images dominate the text, Proverbs ends with a lengthy poem praising women (Proverbs 31:10-31). The image presented of womanhood is matronly and dignified:

> Strength and dignity are her clothing, and she laughs at the time to come. She opens her mouth with wisdom, and the teaching of kindness is on her tongue. (31:25-26)

Even by modern standards, the Jewish woman of this ancient poem had important roles to play other than housekeeping and child rearing:

> She considers a field and buys it; with the fruit of her hands she plants a vineyard. She girds herself with strength, and makes her arms strong. She perceives that her merchandise is profitable. (31:16-18)

Apparently, the basic education of children was the responsibility of the family. Perhaps as children grew older and abilities began to emerge, their formal education took different routes. Some might have become, in effect, apprentices to older siblings or adults within the broader family structure. Some, with the proper abilities, would have been trained to serve the monarchy. All Hebrew males might have gone to the Temple to study, but since the priesthood was an inherited right, only the members of certain tribes received formal education related to the service of priests. Regardless of occupation, gender or community status, the book of Proverbs represents a common body of wisdom and instruction that all Hebrews would have been taught. And, just as in other cultures, that body of knowledge would have been well developed and transmitted to the young through the oral tradition for centuries before anyone put it in writing and before there was anything called a school or a textbook.

For the sake of establishing a common ground of virtue, let us examine the wisdom offered in Proverbs as it relates to the main virtues taught by Socrates (justice, courage, moderation, friendship and wisdom). There are a small number of statements in Proverbs about moderation. The book of Ecclesiastes places far more emphasis on moderation and may have been placed in the Bible immediately after Proverbs to balance what often seems a heavy-handed view on moral instruction. The few statements in Proverbs about moderation are more humorous than profound:

> If you have found honey, eat only enough for you, or else, having too much, you will vomit it. (25:16)
>
> Let your foot be seldom in your neighbor's house, otherwise the neighbor will become weary of you and hate you. (25:17)

Friendship is a more significant theme in Proverbs. The text often emphasizes the importance of friendship and provides practical tips on how to maintain it:

> One who forgives an affront fosters friendship, but one who dwells on disputes will alienate a friend. (17: 9)
>
> Some friends play at friendship but a true friend sticks closer than one's nearest kin. (18:24)
>
> Make no friends with those given to anger, and do not associate with hotheads, or you may learn their ways and entangle yourself in a snare. (22:24)

Wisdom is the dominant theme in Proverbs. In a conceptual sense, wisdom is a broad term that encompasses knowledge, insight, and judgment. A wise person possesses useful knowledge, has insight into the nature of people and event, and exercises good judgment. The book closely connects wisdom with these and other related concepts:[17]

> Get *wisdom*; get *insight*: do not forget, nor turn away from the words of my mouth. (22:24)
>
> Does not *wisdom* call, and does not *understanding* raise her voice? (8:1)
>
> I, *wisdom*, live with *prudence*, and I attain *knowledge* and *discretion*. (3:7)

The book of Proverbs offers useful advice about the conduct of the wise and the way to wisdom:

> Do not be wise in your own eye. (3:7)
>
> ... the wise listen to advice. (12:15)
>
> The wise are cautious and turn away from evil, ... (14:16)

A student of Proverbs cannot be mistaken about the importance, the usefulness and the beauty of wisdom:

> ... the fountain of wisdom is a gushing stream. (18:4)

> ... for wisdom is better than jewels, and all that you may desire cannot compare with her. (8:11)

Justice is also a major theme in Proverbs and was an area in which young males were in particular need of training, since, as they grew into adulthood and became the heads of families or "elders," they would be expected to take "their places at the city gate to mediate disputes and render judgments for the common good."[18] Proverbs contains a number of legal principles necessary to establish justice. For example:

> To impose a fine on the innocent is not right, ... (17:26)

> The one who first states a case seems right, until the other comes and cross-examines. (18:17)

> These also are sayings of the wise: Partiality in judging is not good. (24:23)

Proverbs offers considerably less practical advice on the virtue of courage than on justice, but statements extolling the value of courage are in the text:

> The wicked flee when no one pursues, but the righteous are as bold as a lion. (28:1)

The following passage about courage and justice leads to some conclusions about the intended audience of much of the wisdom in Proverbs:

> If you faint in the day of adversity, your strength being small; if you hold back from rescuing those taken away to death, those who go staggering to the slaughter; if you say, "Look, we did not know this"—does not he who weighs the heart perceive it? Does not he who keeps watch over your soul know it? And will he not repay all according to their deeds? (24:10-12)

This passage suggests that establishing a just society will require wisdom and courage, and that claiming ignorance, in the end, will not relieve us of our responsibility or guilt. In the two questions at the end of the passage, the absence of words like God, LORD, king, or judge is quite striking. Surely, the sage here is referring to the LORD, in much the way the phrase "fear of the LORD" is so often used in Proverbs:

> The fear of the LORD is the beginning of knowledge; fools despise wisdom and instruction. (1:7)

> The fear of the LORD prolongs life, but the years of the wicked will be short. (10:27)

Perhaps it could be argued that the phrase "the fear of the LORD" is synonymous with reverence, or reverence for the LORD. But the translators preferred the word "fear" to the word "reverence" because fear is closest in meaning to what the context of the book is suggesting. The sages, the ancient teachers of the Israelite children, used a pedagogical strategy that teachers and parents often attempt to use today, particularly with older children and adolescents—fear. Those who were not attentive to wisdom and instruction were destined for "the pit" or "Sheol," or, more familiarly, hell:

> For the wise the path of life leads upward, in order to avoid Sheol below. (15:24)

> One who walks in integrity will be safe, but whoever follows crooked ways will fall into the Pit. (28:18)

This point is important for several reasons. First, though there are many, important similarities between the teaching of Socrates and the book of Proverbs, the differences between the two are less of philosophy or religion, and more of intended audience. Socrates believed in the Greek gods and held that piety was an important quality of character. But Socrates, at least as he is known through Plato's *Republic*, offers teaching to a more restricted and older audience than the intended audience of Proverbs. Socrates' teaching was intended for the male, ruling class of the Greek city-state. The pedagogy of Socrates is one that would be effective with older, more mature students. Socrates treats his students as his equals. The Socratic approach to teaching is a meaningful term today and is, sometimes, used with younger students. But the direct, often heavy-handed, fear-evoking approach of Proverbs is still used by parents and teachers when children challenge and disrupt the order.

Blended into the beauty and wisdom of Proverbs is also some of the desperation of parents of stubborn teenagers, of teachers whose children are prone to inattention, laziness and disrespect. A common structure of the proverbial sentence is a set of parallel clauses in which the word "but" establishes the antithetical relationship between the first and the second clause. After making our point about the right thing to do, most of us cannot resist the temptation of follow-up with a warning about the bad:

> Whoever is slow to anger has great understanding, but one who has a hasty temper exalts folly. (14:29)
>
> A gracious woman gets honor, but she who hates virtue is covered with shame. (11:16)

Particularly when children's behavior angers us and makes us fearful for what the future holds for them, we are prone to instruct and warn of the "bad." Proverbs offers heavy armament for such times. It gives as much attention to the vices as to the virtues. It establishes a deep and rich vocabulary for understanding both sides of moral behavior, the good and the bad. A precise count of the vices named is difficult because of overlapping meanings, but there are at least seventy different words used in Proverbs for naming the vices, from adultery to wrath. Some of the words used to admonish the learners are words of anger, words like "fool," "stupid," "hothead," and "lazybones." The word "fool" and its derivatives are used ninety times in the NRSV!

Clearly, much of the content of Proverbs was intended for children and adolescents. The vocabulary, the sentence structure and the implied instructional strategies of many passages suggest that some of the sages would not fit the archetypal image of wise men as people who live in isolation in the wilderness, the temple, or the king's court. In Proverbs, the wise were people deeply involved in the lives of their children, their neighbors and the village. They were more than scholars and community leaders; they were parents and teachers who knew their words were not always heeded. They knew that children have difficulty resisting the temptation of whatever provides pleasure. They knew that adolescents seem destined to deny authority and to regard their parents as hopelessly out-of-date. They threatened and pleaded for their children's attention. The words "rebuke" and "reproof" are used nineteen times, with the usual suggestion being that wise children accept being rebuked.

> A wise child loves discipline, but a scoffer does not listen to rebuke. (13:1)

> Poverty and disgrace are for the one who ignores instruction, but one who heeds reproof is honored. (13:18)

When a verbal rebuke failed, there was a next step recommended, the rod. "The rod" appears in Proverbs five times. Its role as an element of instruction is unmistakable:

> Those who spare the rod hate their children, but those who love them are diligent to discipline them. (13:24)

> Folly is bound up in the heart of a boy, but the rod of discipline drives it far away. (22:15)

This reference to "spanking" is present, but it is not a major theme. Three of the five occurrences are in chapters 22 and 23. Most of the different collections within the book make no reference to physical punishment as an element of discipline. Of the twelve verses in the book that use the word discipline, only three connect it to "the rod."

Though the child-rearing strategies and sometimes the language of Proverbs may seem archaic the basic ideas are universal and timeless—even the ones about heeding a reproof. This ancient text is a poetic document that defines in detail the good and the bad. It is often specific and concrete and was intended to offer wisdom to all Hebrews, regardless of age, tribe or gender. Though the style and intended audience make the book of Proverbs a very different text when compared to the teaching of Socrates, the anonymous sages of Proverbs share with Socrates a common body of moral principles and a common view that wisdom is transmitted from one generation to the next by instruction and by the desire for learning and self-improvement.

CONFUCIUS AND HIS VIEW OF CHARACTER

Like most of the ancient sages, the identity of Confucius is blurred by multiple legends and by the interpretations of and elaborations on his teaching. He lived slightly before the time of Socrates (551-479 B.C.E.).[19] During his life, Confucius was a wandering teacher who sought work in the courts of various Chinese rulers. Eventually, he became highly regarded as one who could train "the sons of gentlemen in the virtues proper to a member of the ruling class."[20] After his death, students and disciples preserved and added to

According to Waley, the teaching of Confucius was often not accepted in the Chinese courts, causing frustration and hardship and sending Confucius on his travels from state to state in search a of ruler who would embrace his teaching. Though he sought the status of statesman and diplomat, there is no historical evidence that Confucius ever achieved it. It was not until after his death that he was elevated to the level of Divine Sage.[21]

As a teacher, Confucius took no credit for the knowledge and wisdom he disseminated. As written in the *Analects*:

> The Master said, I have "transmitted what was taught to me without making up anything of my own." I have been faithful to and loved the Ancients. (Bk. VII:1)

The goal Confucius set for himself was to impart knowledge that had been passed down to him by ancient sages and to form the character of his students according to the traditions of the past. The culture of his time was much in need of a steadying, moral force. He lived in a period of Chinese history marked by "political corruption, warfare, disintegrating society, and declining personal standards."[22] In the latter years of his life, Confucius found some measure of satisfaction and public stature. After his death, for 1600 years, the *Analects* existed as an important scripture among other scripture. However, in the twelfth century C.E., during the Sung dynasty, "it became a school-book, and finally not merely a school-book, but the school-book, basis of all education."[23] As we see by some of the proverbs that will follow, the wisdom Confucius offered was practical and was intended to help establish peace, order and justice in the family, community and the King's court.

Confucius' character foundation has endured for over 2400 years and has profoundly influenced the moral fabric of a fourth of the world's population, but his basic text is a challenge for western readers. As with the book of Proverbs, new readers can pick out proverbial "gems," but it is considerably more challenging to see the unifying themes. The *Analects* of Confucius consists of twenty short "books," many of which were probably written by disciples rather than Confucius himself. In the book's apparent lack of structure, there is similarity between the *Analects* and Proverbs. The vocabulary, sentence structure, and themes suggest several voices that emphasize different aspects of character. The wisdom is proverbial, therefore usually concise and poetic. The proverbs often seem randomly ordered and are occasionally repetitious. Confucius, the sage, composer and compiler of usually concise and poetic. The proverbs often seem randomly ordered and are occasionally repetitious. Confucius, the sage, composer and compiler of wisdom, like the unknown editor of Proverbs, made little use of anything resembling an organizing system in which proverbs about a particular theme would be placed together. Though sometimes a Master or King is cited by name as the source of a saying, the idea of systematically referencing information would have to wait a couple of thousand years. No chapter titles or headings orient the reader to a text structure or provide any clue as to the direction of the ideas. Also, as with some passages in Proverbs, a reader of the *Analects* who has no prior knowledge of the cultural context will have difficulty unlocking the meaning and significance of some proverbs.

According to Jeffrey Wattles, in his book on the universality of the golden rule, Confucian teachings describe the nature of five relationships: father and son, husband and wife, older brother and younger brother, emperor and minister, and friend and friend.[24] If these relationships were expressed in democratic and gender-free terms, they would encompass most of the important relationships of a lifetime. As Wattles points out, in the time of Confucius these relationships involved acting properly as a superior or a subordinate, with the exception of the friend to friend relationship.[25] The broader body of literature that developed from the teaching of Confucius and his disciples may fully describe these five relationships; but in the *Analects* Confucius primarily addresses the relationship of ruler to subjects, sons to fathers, and friends to friends. The following are examples of proverbial wisdom from Confucius about these relationships:

> In serving his father and mother, a man may gently remonstrate with them. But if he sees that he has failed to change their opinion, he should resume an attitude of deference and not thwart them. (Bk. IV:18)

> Master Yu said, Those who in private life behave well towards their parents and elder brothers, in public life seldom show a disposition to resist the authority of their superiors. (Bk. I:2)

> The Master said, He whose wisdom brings him into power and who has Goodness to secure it, if he has not dignity wherewith to approach the common people, they will not respect him. (Bk. XV:32)

> The Master said, A country of a thousand war-chariots cannot be administered unless the ruler attends strictly to business, punctually observes his promises, is economical in expenditure, shows affection towards his subjects in general, and uses the labour of the peasantry only at the proper times of year. (Bk. I:5)

> The Master said, the Good Person collects friends about him and through these friends promotes Goodness. (Bk. XII:24)
>
> That friends should come to one from afar, is this not after all delightful? (Bk.I:1)

Confucius used the term *tao* (literally, "the road, a path, a way") to refer to the way in which something good was accomplished.[26] In later Confucian writing, *tao* came to have a more formal meaning, referring to a method or principle which guided good behavior, thus "The Way,"[27] the habitual practices that form good character. The Way is both a spiritual and practical concept, a reference to the path to good families, friendships and communities. In the *Analects*, Confucius uses *tao* (or The Way, as moderns express it) as a broad term that encompasses the living wisdom of the ancient ones:

> The Master said, The gentleman, in his plans, thinks of the Way; he does not think how he is going to earn a living. (Bk. XV:31)

But the phrase, if not the formal concept, is not unique to Confucius or the Chinese. It is also common in the teaching of Buddha,[28] whose scriptures originate in India:

> How can a troubled mind understand the way?[29]

and is an expression that occurs in both the Old Testament:

> Hear, my child, and be wise, and direct your mind in the way. (Prov. 23:19)

and the New Testament:

> Jesus said to him, "I am the way, and the truth, and the life. No one comes to the Father except through me." (John 14:6)

How do the major themes of Confucius compare to the commonly recognized virtues of Socrates and the book of Proverbs? The wisdom we find in the teaching of Confucius would certainly support the important elements of good character taught by Socrates: justice, courage, moderation, friendship and wisdom. In the *Analects*, Confucius does not speak often or directly about justice, certainly not to the extent of either Socrates or Proverbs. But the value of a just community is unmistakable:

> He who is just is the joy of the people. (Bk. XX:1)

Confucius does not often speak directly about courage; but the importance of courage in following The Way is clearly implied:

> Meet resentment with upright dealing and meet inner power with inner power. (Bk. XIV: 36)

> The Master said, a gentleman can withstand hardships; it is only a small man who, when submitted to hardship, is swept off his feet. (Bk. XV: 1)

However, courage is a character trait that may not be desirable in the extreme.

> Love of courage without love of learning degenerates into turbulence. (Bk. XVII: 8)

The word moderation is not used in Waley's translation, but some of the proverbs (like the one above about courage) point to a moderate path of behavior about several matters:

> The Master said, Pleasure not carried to the point of debauch; grief not carried to the point of self-injury. (Bk. III: 20)

> The Master fished with a line but not a net; when fowling he did not aim at a roosting bird. (Bk. VII: 26)

As Wattles points out, the relationship among friends was an important Confucian theme:

> Master K'ung said, There are three sorts of friendship that are profitable, and three sorts that are harmful. Friendship with the upright, with the true-to-death and with those who have heard much is profitable. Friendship with the obsequious, friendship with those who are good at accommodating their principles, friendship with those who are clever at talk is harmful. (Bk. XVI: 5)

The word wisdom does not often occur in the *Analects*. As with so many important character themes, Confucius did not often speak directly about it. His approach to wisdom was practical and metaphorical, but it was not direct.

Whereas the sages of Proverbs seemed obsessed with naming and defining over and again the virtues and vices, Confucius was more prone to make insightful observations about wise human behavior which required the reader to infer the important meaning. One of his most direct statements about wisdom is the following:

> The Master said, He whose wisdom brings him into power, needs Goodness to secure that power. (Bk. XV: 32)

Beyond this idea, Confucius mostly spoke about wisdom by using other words. One of the most commonly occurring words in the *Analects* is goodness. In my database that contains ninety-seven Confucian proverbs,[30] the word goodness is found twelve times. Here is a sampling of how he used the term:

> The Master said, *Goodness* is more to the people than water and fire. (Bk. XV: 34)
>
> The Master said, It is *Goodness* that gives a neighborhood its beauty. (Bk. IV: 1).
>
> The Master said, *Goodness* cannot be obtained till what is difficult has been duly done. (Bk. VI: 20)

Like the sages from the other cultures, Confucius knew that obtaining wisdom required the work of learning. He says, in the *Analects*, that he was not born with wisdom, that he did not receive it by inspiration, that he had to learn it, and that it took him fifty years:

> The Master said, I for my part am not one of those who have innate knowledge. I am simply one who loves the past and who is diligent in investigating it. (Bk. VII: 19)

Many of the Confucian proverbs, fourteen of the ninety-seven in my database, speak directly or indirectly to the value of learning. Again, here is a sample:

> The Master said, I once spent a whole day without food and a whole night without sleep in order to meditate. It was no use. It is better to *learn*. (Bk. XV: 30)

> The Master said, Little ones, Why is it that none of you *study* the Songs? For the Songs will help you to incite people's emotions, to observe their feelings, to keep company, to express your grievances. ... Moreover, they will *widen your acquaintance* with the names of birds, beasts, plants and trees. (Bk. XVII: 9)

> Love of uprightness without *love of learning* degenerates into harshness. (Bk. XVII: 8)

Similarities among Confucius, Socrates and *Proverbs* have been noted: Wisdom, friendship, goodness, the desire to learn, and justice are at the center of good character. The journey that leads to these qualities is not a singular journey. Good character cannot develop in solitude. It is nurtured in families or communities of good character. In the absence of family or friends, the strength of character of a hermit cannot be known. Both the *Analects* of Confucius and Proverbs offer much practical wisdom about how to establish and maintain those relationships. As Confucius described the many aspects of goodness, he pointed his disciples and future readers along the Way to good relationships.

Any of the three sources of wisdom discussed here would provide an excellent moral guide to a person of any culture or time. But the combined wisdom of all three sources offers a more complete and far-reaching view of character. The directness and detail of Proverbs may be more accessible to children. Though the New Revised Standard Version (1989) is used here, Today's English Version (1976) offers a translation of the Bible that uses more contemporary English vocabulary and sentence structure and might be the version of Proverbs best suited for children and teenagers. Much of the wisdom of Socrates and Confucius is quite understandable to older children and teenagers. Adults routinely underestimate the intellectual ability and moral reasoning power of children and teenagers.

This discussion is but a small dip into the pool of ancient wisdom. There are, for example, sixty-five other books of the Protestant Bible, the other Socratic dialogues of Plato, the Koran, the Buddhist scriptures, the writings of sages like Aristotle and Lao-tzu, and the multitude of collected proverbs from almost every culture of the world. There is no lack of wisdom to be read and digested. Unfortunately, wisdom literature is so rarely read that we are mostly unaware of the universality of our understanding of good character. In this brief glimpse of proverbial wisdom from three different cultures we can see the common fabric of goodness that is spread across humanity, which brings us back to the beginning thesis: if we examine the virtues taught by our cultural ancestors, we find a common ground of virtue and see that formal education, what we call schooling, has always included character development—not religion, but the values, behaviors and habits that represent goodness around the globe. People of various cultures differ in many ways, from the food they eat, the clothes they wear, the languages they speak, to the gods they worship. However, though the words used to define and describe good character may differ, the fundamental meanings of those words are much the same.

THE MODERN SCHOOL AND THE CHARACTER OF OUR CHILDREN

How do we make the leap of 2,500 years, from Socrates, *Proverbs* and Confucius to American public schools in the twenty-first century? First, we should admit that secular schooling has the potential to be a force—not *the* force, but *a* force—in shaping character. Teachers could use the wisdom literature from various cultures to engage students in ethical discussions, writing, and art. Excerpts from Proverbs, the *Analects*, *The Republic*, or other sources could be used in reading, literature and history classes and could occasionally be used appropriately in other subject areas. Public school teachers cannot teach religion, but can use scriptural literature as instructional material. Proverbial wisdom might be particularly useful; the variety, brevity, and range of sophistication make proverbs convenient for almost any grade level or subject area. Ultimately, proverbial wisdom touches everything and everybody.

Character education does not need a special name, time or place in the curriculum. It is already there—unless there has been a lapse in cultural memory. Character education is present in good instruction about many subjects. For example, history is about the conflicts among communities and the search for justice. It is the story of how the virtues and vices have been played on the human stage. History will teach character.

Reading good literature provides exposure to events and behaviors that determine character. Good literature begins early with the disobedience and punishment of *Peter Rabbit* and leads toward the moral dilemma of Huckleberry Finn's companionship with Jim, the run-away slave. Literature is about love and death, and all that comes before, between and after. Good books will teach character when students read, discuss and write about the universal dilemmas faced by the characters. It is demanding work, but when knowledgeable and able teachers hold their students to high expectations of disciplined study, good character is being formed.

No matter what we call it, no matter if we are direct or indirect, our efforts to use school to shape the character of our children will not succeed if the character of our school is not good. Elements of schooling other than the curriculum influence character development. The organization and the administration of the school affects character development, either positively or negatively. The campus must be a safe and just place. Parents need to support teachers and principals who work to create orderly, effective schools. But the educators must be wise in the use of power. The children and teenagers must perceive the school as a fair place—a place which does not show favoritism to skin color, gender, or ability.

Is this a tall order for a school system serving millions of children of various ethnic and economic backgrounds? Can we realistically expect teachers to have the identity and demeanor of Socrates or Confucius? No, the ancient sages are models for what a teacher might be, but they were elite teachers in societies where only the children of the elite went to school. Ancient Greece had no need of a million Socrates. Whether it be false dreaming or not, American society at the end of the twentieth century is built on the assumption, dating back to the 1640s and the Massachusetts Bay Colony, that wherever there is a community, there should be a school. Now we must have not a small number of teachers for the selected few but millions of teachers for a nation of schools. The best of those teachers will approach the power and influence of Socrates, at least in the eyes of their students. The rest of the teachers will have to work at sagehood as diligently as Confucius had to work at learning. As written texts have accumulated over the millennia, perhaps wisdom is being buried by information. Perhaps, to teach the good, we will have to unbury it. Do we have the will, the self-discipline, and the foresight to do that? The wisdom cited above should provide a source of hope and inspiration. The good (the way, the moral, the ethical) is not elusive. It has been explained in many languages with memorable words, metaphors and sayings. It was there before we had the capacity to save it in a written form. Confucius and the other wise men said so, that they were not making up the wisdom, they were simply recording what they had learned from the ancient ones. In one sense, nothing has changed in 2500 years. If we want to understand the good, whether we are teachers, parents or students, we must seek it, attend to it, and convert the words into habits.

NOTES

1. K. Ryan & M. Cooper, *Those Who Can, Teach* (New York: Houghton Mifflin, 1998), 333.
2. Joel Spring, *The American School, 1642-1985* (New York: Longman, 1986), 141.
3. Ibid.
4. C.D.C. Reeve, Introduction. to Plato, *The Republic*, trans. G.M.A. Grube, rev. C.D.C. Reeve (Indianapolis: Hackett, 1992), xii.
5. For the purpose of this analysis, I am relying on standard English translations of the primary texts. The specific translations are identified in the notes.
6. Plato, *The Republic*. All references to *The Republic* are from this text.
7. Reeve, xvii.
8. Plato, 451c-471c.
9. Italics are mine to emphasize the connection between the proverbial statements and the five virtues.
10. S. Hels, "Introduction to Wisdom Literature," in *Old Testament Wisdom,* ed. M.E. Williams (Nashville: Abingdon, 1994), 14.
11. R.E. Friedman, *Who Wrote the Bible?* (New York: Summit, 1987), 213.
12. All biblical quotations in this text are from the New Revised Standard Version.
13. M.E. Williams, *Old Testament Wisdom,* 26.
14. Ibid.
15. Ibid.
16. Luke 2:41-52.
17. The italics are mine to show the connections among the key words.
18. Williams, 26.
19. Jeffrey Wattles, *The Golden Rule* (New York: Oxford, 1996), 15.
20. Arthur Waley, intro. to *The Analects of Confucius*, trans. Arthur Waley (New York: Random House, 1938), 13-17. All references attributed to Confucius appear in this text.
21. Ibid.
22. Wattles, 15.
23. Waley, 72.
24. Wattles, 15-16.
25. Ibid., 16.
26. Waley, 23.
27. The capitalization of "w" in "Way" is the result of modern, western orthography.
28. In Buddhist scripture, the Way is referred to as the *Dharma.*
29. Quoted in J. Kornfield, *The Teachings of Buddha* (Boston: Shambhala, 1996), 4.
30. A personal database, including about 1500 proverbs from many different sources.

QUESTIONS FOR DISCUSSION

1. What roles should parents and teachers assume in developing protective boundaries for children? What would Socrates suggest?

2. Those who support developmental and age appropriate curricula would have no problem with Socrates' ideas on educating the young. How do these practices develop character: use of play, avoidance of abrasive methods, and assessing individual interest?

3. Other than fear of the Lord, what strategies could the modern teacher use to share the wisdom of Proverbs with his or her students? Is the sharing of such wisdom separable from religious instruction?

4. In both Socrates and Proverbs, what wisdom is being transmitted to the younger generation by their elders ? How are the desire for learning and the quest for self-improvement best communicated from generation to generation?

5. Confucius relates wisdom to goodness. Are there any significant differences between goodness and wisdom? How could Confucius' "Way" be used to design a character education program?

6. Where might Socrates, Proverbs, and Confucius fit into teacher preparation programs? What should teachers know about Proverbs, the *Analects*, and *The Republic*?

7. Who or what teaches character?

8. In paragraph one of the essay, Hemphill asks, "Is character development within the realm of responsibility for public schools?" What do you think?

ATTENDING BEAUTY:
THE INHERENT ETHIC OF PARTICIPATION IN ART

Ray Martin

ABSTRACT

The changing language of visual art has enabled artists to join directly in the discussion of the good. This essay explains how choosing to participate in beauty begins with pleasure and leads to love. An education in beauty is explored as a moral responsibility and a powerful gift for the elevation of both the individual and society.

Form is the external expression of internal meaning.
—Wassily Kandinsky

We all know that Art is not Truth. Art is a lie that makes us realize truth, at least the truth that is given us to understand. The artist must know the manner whereby to convince others of the truthfulness of his lies.
——Pablo Picasso

Pablo Picasso exhorts his fellow artists to master their craft because he believes art to be a formal language capable of expressing truth in an "instantaneous unity," whole and recognizable at once, as compared to other formal languages which exist within a chronological time frame. For example, the readers of a novel or viewers of a film may only evaluate the full meaning of these forms after the experience. Removed from the immediacy of reading and viewing, they "re-member" the events in a residuum. The great Russian abstractionist Wassily Kandinsky wrote of encountering a painting as a visceral experience "consist[ing] of sudden illuminations, like lightning, of explosions, which burst like a fireworks in the heavens, strewing a whole bouquet of different shining stars about itself. These illuminations show new perspectives in a blinding light, new truths."[1]

The difficulty in translating such instantaneous insights from the visual form to the written word may help explain why artists are hesitant to approach the field of ethics. Nevertheless, this essay will attempt to explain how the visual arts came to be involved in a discussion of the "good," why participation in the beautiful is morally elevating, and what benefits are inherent in an education in beauty.

ARTISTS AS PARTICIPANTS IN ETHICS

In non-Western societies there is often no distinguishing word for "art" or "artist." For many of these cultures the tasks of making visual images, dances, songs and theatrical performances fall to the shamans of the community. These singular persons have the triune tasks of healing the sick, communicating the will of the sacred powers, and creating supernaturally useful images and objects for the benefit of their communities. Their "art" has moral authority for these societies because it serves the community's religious and secular authorities through the enchanting illustration of shared moral precepts, not because it stems from the shaman's particular conscience.

For the greater part of the last two millennia Western artists also had little or no independent moral position in their society. They might make works of great moral fervor and subtlety, but they were usually working for powers in the Church. For example, no matter how much personal passion a medieval artist brought to a fresco, contemporaries viewing it would regard the Biblical story—not the artist himself or his illustration of it—as the source of authority. Even during the zenith of the Italian Renaissance in 1500, signature geniuses Michelangelo and Leonardo da Vinci were bound not to exceed subtle embellishments of ecclesiastically approved religious and moral conventions. The "lie that makes us realize truth," as Picasso called it, belonged to the greater social institution, not the questing individual. This was as true for the Christian artist as it had been for the tribal shaman.

But during the nineteenth century, a cataclysmic change occurred for the European image-maker. The lessening cultural role of religion left the artist bereft of his traditional motif. Not only was the Christian story ceasing to exist as subject and economic fodder for the artist, but the camera had been invented. Although the "magic lantern" robbed many an artist of a livelihood by capturing surface reality more accurately and swiftly than any painter, it also liberated the artist to focus on issues other than recording outward information.

When God and mimesis (the latter being Plato's accusation of art's limitation) were removed from the pedestal, many artists found only themselves to place on the perch. At times they accepted this newfound loftiness haltingly, at other times defiantly. Without the demands of representing cultural iconographics or recording the natural world, individual spiritual exploration and personal moral searching became the direct subject matter for visual creators. As a result, it was inevitable that the recognizable world would grow indistinct and eventually disappear altogether. In the twentieth century, artists such as Kandinsky and Mark Rothko came to hope their use of shapes, colors and compositional placements would serve as visual "blueprints" for spiritual harmony on the part of their audience.

Today it seems naive to expect the mere viewing of an art work to bring meaningful change to a person or society. Yet, the passive pleasure of aesthetic experience, by its generative nature, can evoke an active involvement in the beautiful. Further, this involvement has the potential to imbue the participant with a beneficent love.

ART AS PARTICIPATION IN BEAUTY

The dual nature of passive and active involvement in beauty is described by Robert Grudin, noted writer in the study of aesthetics.

> If beauty results from our insight into the integrity or fitness of phenomena, what are the effects of such insight? We may describe two sorts of effect: *pleasure and love.* Pleasure is the passive effect of beauty, the receptive sensation that, at the moment of insight or recognition, expresses itself, complete with adrenal burst, in wonder or laughter or tears. Love, on the other hand, is the active effect of beauty: the will to repeat or increase pleasure by participating in beauty as fully as possible. Thus the people who are most capable of insight are most avid in their pursuit of chances to exercise it.[2]

There is a Zen saying that Westerners are so busy *doing* that they never take time to *be*. Grudin's definition of insight into beauty incorporates both states as mutually beneficial. Being receptive to beauty inspires the will to *do*.

Cataloguing the visual facts of an observed experience does not fulfill the cycle from pleasure to love. I may walk through the forest behind my mother's house and respond to the wonder of sensory stimulations there. The pines whisper like an ocean in my ear, punctuated by the trilling of a songbird. The sun traces light around the silhouettes of needles on the forest floor. Warm and fragrant air gently coaxes my skin and nostrils to continue on the trail. Dazzling, harmonious colors of flower, earth and air dance before my eyes. At this point I am filled with joy at the perceptual pleasures received. But the insight into beauty is not yet complete. Aesthetic experience begins with a sudden change in my frame of mind. I begin to look at the landscape not only as spectator but with an artist's eye. I form, in my mind, a "picture" of the landscape. In this picture none of the observed qualities are forgotten or effaced. Even the strongest and most powerful artistic imagination cannot create a new world *ex nihilo*, out of nothing.

But when the artist approaches nature, all its elements assume a new shape. Artistic imagination and contemplation do not give us the essence of dead physical things with mute sense-qualities. They give us a world of moving and living form—a balance of lights and shadow, of rhythms and melodies, of lines and contours, of patterns and designs. This evoking of beauty fills us with unspeakable delight and seems to renew the world. Such immersion in forming, such active participation in beauty resembles other sorts of love in every respect, except that it has no personal object or physical goal.[3] The full participation in beauty develops a passion for what George Santayana refers to as the "quality of a thing... . Beauty is a value, that is, it is not a perception of a matter of fact or a relation: it is an emotion, an affection of our volitional and appreciative nature."[4]

Quality is defined as degree of excellence, that which is characteristic or noble about a thing. This was known in classical Greek thought as *aretē*, virtue, and is considered worthwhile in itself. Assessing the worth of a thing, defining traits of its being, or appreciating its loftiness, can only come from a reflective appreciation, involving both the object of attention and the assessor. We cannot understand beauty without participating in it, or participate in it without subsuming its principles. As we form art, art forms us.

In any great work of art the relation of detail to the larger composition is critical. This is what formalist critics such as Clement Greenberg have called "significant form," and it provides a model of what one would wish of a just world, in which every detail had its right, proper, and exciting place in some larger scheme. This concept mirrors Plato's emphasis on virtue, which he considers akin to beauty: "Virtue makes the soul harmonious, as beauty orders the elements of a face or a scene. Even Plato's ideal republic involves the aesthetic notion of harmoniously organized parts."[5] A great work of art rarely leads toward any particular moral conclusion but instead opens the mind to a kind of aesthetic reverie, which includes the sensation that here, at last, is something sufficient—as life would be in a better world. Thus, through devotion to purely aesthetic success, an artist can convey intense moral truth.

ART AS EDUCATION IN BEAUTY

An education omitting the arts speaks only to the external, physical world of facts. Understanding is incomplete without insight into the emotional, intuitive and spiritual truths of internal reality. The arts reveal these truths and imbue function with meaning. Of all the elements of learning, the perception of beauty is at once the most delightful and the most suggestive of an underlying principle that unites the disciplines. True teachers always convey the sense that the communication of an art demands of the student not only effort and attention but cathartic psychological change. To learn is not merely to accumulate data; it is to rebuild one's world. The artist who rejects teaching rejects the ethical imperative demanded by the participation in beauty.[6]

I always begin my classes with an invitation to the students to *attend* class during the semester. "Attend" derives from the Latin *attendere*, "to reach toward, to stretch." I believe art can be used for the vital function of awakening the perceptual and creative capacities in the individual consciousness. Grudin makes the point even more emphatically:

> If beauty is a necessary factor in a natural relationship, if it follows inevitably from the accurate perception of form, if it inspires pleasure and love, unifies reason and emotion, and provokes continued achievement, then all true education is education in beauty. Excellence of mind itself, rightly conceived, is expertise in beauty; creativity is wise love.[7]

How might we guide another in the path to "wise love"? In *The Education of Little Tree,* a five-year-old Cherokee boy queried his grandmother regarding the meaning of life and death. The old woman spoke of the existence of two "minds." One was a "body-living" mind concerned with the necessities of everyday existence. The second "mind" was inhabited by the spirit. If a person focused only on developing the first consciousness, then:

That's how you become dead people, Granma said you could easy spot dead people. She said dead people when they looked at a woman saw nothing but dirty; when they looked at other people they saw nothing but bad; when they looked at a tree they saw nothing but lumber and profit, never *beauty*. Granma said they was dead people walking around. Granma said that the spirit mind was like any other muscle. If you used it it got bigger and stronger. She said the only way it could get that way was using it to understand, but you couldn't open the door to it until you quit being greedy and such with your body mind. The understanding commenced to take up, and the more you tried to understand, the bigger it got. Natural, she said, *understand* and *love* was the same thing; except folks went at it back'ards too many times, trying to pretend they loved things when they didn't understand them. Which can't be done.[8]

"Understanding" for Granma echoes the Cherokee concept of *Orinda*, right relationship. Deciding to participate in the beauty of the tree begins the journey toward recognizing one's own place in an interdependent universe. Such involvement leads to a knowing love.

Art for children is primarily a means of expression, a way of exploring and explaining the self as a dynamic being, a way that helps them recognize their place in an interdependent universe. Art becomes a language of thought, of learning, and a way to search for answers that words cannot adequately supply. For a child, art-making is an external process serving as a vehicle for internal progress on the pathway to the self. In contrast, for many adults in our society, art has taken on quite different meanings: museums, pictures hanging on walls, full-color reproductions, and a general feeling of an activity that is removed from the "body mind" of making a living. Art for many adults is limited to that same "body mind" that produces some sort of art *product* for consumption or purchase. At what age is it appropriate to educate children to the transition in understanding regarding the purpose of art for adults? Should we re-examine the possibility that a "childlike" hunger to participate in beauty has the potential to be vital to an individual's life and healthy for a society? As children grow into adulthood, could they be educated through art into the beauty of "spirit mind"?

For example, every person in a traditional Balinese village has two "jobs." Each family member is a gardener and also an artist. Every grandparent has taught every son and daughter, in exquisite detail, how to grow bounteous, luscious food and flowers. Every grandparent has taught every son and daughter how to carve, draw and paint beautiful, intricate images full of visual magic. These sons and daughters have taught their children the same knowledge. No one in traditional Bali has a concept that he or she is *not* an artist.

as "outsiders." They are thought of as eccentrics who may be imbued by a vaguely understood magic known as "talent," but have only token usefulness in practical terms. This is a dangerous misconception. Until each person accepts the invitation proffered by the pleasure and love available from immersion in beauty, he or she is at risk for the spiritual fatigue and atrophy spoken of in *Little Tree*. This malady inevitably extends to and poisons the greater society. On the other hand, by actively participating in beauty one accepts a healing gift as well as a moral responsibility. Such a choice invites joy into the human experience and begins the process of re-enchanting the world.

NOTES

1. Wassily Kandinsky, "Reminiscences," in *Modern Artists on Art*, ed. Robert L. Herbert (Englewood Cliffs, NJ: Prentice-Hall, Inc. 1964).
2. Robert Grudin, *The Grace of Great Things* (New York: Ticknor & Fields, 1990).
3. George Santayana, *The Sense of Beauty*, (Cambridge, MA: Harvard University Press, 1896); reprinted in *A World of Ideas,* ed. Lee A. Jacobus (New York: St. Martin's Press, 1983), 541.
4. Robert C. Solomon and Kathleen M. Higgins, *A Short History of Philosophy* (New York: Oxford University Press, 1996).
5. Grudin, 146-154.
6. Grudin, 60-61.
7. Forrest Carter, *The Education of Little Tree* (1976; reprinted London: Rider, 1991). Since its publication, a controversy has arisen regarding the factual authenticity of this work and whether it should be categorized under "biography" or "fiction." This debate has no bearing on my usage here. Once again, this may be an example of Picasso's "lie that tells the truth."

QUESTIONS FOR DISCUSSION

1. Whose interest is reflected in the patronage of the arts in modern society? Do you think the federal government should fund the National Endowment for the Arts?

2. Does one need to think as an artist in order to be delighted by nature and to be taught by nature/beauty? According to the author, how does one acquire the eye of an artist?

3. What does a just world have to do with art? Aesthetic imagination? Beauty?

4. Is beauty universal? Are multiple interpretations justifiable? Where does accurate perception of form fit? Who decides? Can someone perceive art incorrectly?

5. Would we be a better collective society if we were all artists? Is being an artist the path to higher moral ground?

6. What does the example of Balinese society tell us about our own attitudes toward aesthetic beauty and artistic talent?

GAME THEORY, THE CLASSICAL MICROECONOMIC PARADIGM, AND THE ECONOMICS OF ETHICS

Frederick J. Oerther III

ABSTRACT

This paper explores the connection between economics and ethics. We begin by describing the standard behavioral model of economics, the Classical Microeconomic Paradigm (CMP). A number of empirical criticisms have raised the question of whether economic behavior implies that freedom results in outcomes which are bad for society. Attempts by economists to use social welfare functions to defend CMP have been unsuccessful. The CMP has failed to provide a convincing justification of political freedom and economic free markets. Utilizing a branch of mathematics called Game Theory, this paper provides an explanation of how cooperative social institutions evolve, even in situations such as the Prisoner's Dilemma, where the interests of society's members may be directly opposed. Free markets and the ethics of the business community are thus shown to be consistent with the economic model of human behavior and socially beneficial ethical conduct.

GAME THEORY AND ETHICS

The goal of this paper is to provide an ethical foundation for microeconomic science using Game Theory. The effort to modernize economic thought will address criticisms and incorporate insights from the mathematics of Game Theory in order to develop a meaningful connection between economics and ethics. Ultimately, the intention is to provide an ethical foundation for the economics of free markets consistent with the scientific position of classical microeconomics.

Generally speaking, Game Theory is a branch of mathematics which sets up *lemmas* (logical puzzles) to depict various social circumstances. This allows choices faced by social agents (referred to as "players") to be described as *strategies*. Further, Game Theory provides criteria by which agents can anticipate the results of following given strategies; these are described as *payoffs*. In general, Game Theory is a useful tool in economics because it teaches the ethics of social cooperation, and allows an examination of co-operative and coercive behavior within the same logical framework. Game Theory is useful in describing the evolution of *social institutions*, wherein social interactions are ritualized and ultimately stabilized, a state described as *equilibria*. Equilibria are circumstances (i.e., "solutions" to games) in which players have no further incentive to alter their strategy choices, at least in reference to given sets of values/utilities and logical/rational calculations of these players.

The critical insight of Game Theory, which makes it meaningful in an ethics curriculum, is that an individual's payoff depends not only on choices made by that individual but also on the strategic choices employed by the other players in society. Therefore, Game Theory contributes to our understanding about the relationship between individual behavior and community values. Game Theory allows us to make a connection between economics and social ethics. In order to appreciate the contribution that Game Theory can make to exploring the relationship between economics and ethics, a brief digression into the microeconomic paradigm of economic science becomes necessary.

THE CLASSICAL MICROECONOMIC PARADIGM (CMP)

The *Classical Microeconomic Paradigm (CMP)* provides the central insight of economics and hence the primary ethical advocacy of the importance of free markets, which marks the normative position of most economists. In the Classical Microeconomic Paradigm, economists construct a view of human nature that assumes that individuals have subjective values, following the scientific method. A rational economic actor, *homo economicus*, makes decisions on the grounds of utility maximization, subject to constraints imposed by nature and human society. In this view, the mathematics of calculus is used to describe the rational decision-making that economists call *marginal choice*. From the CMP is derived the pure competition model, which describes the economic concept of "efficiency," from which economists have postulated that free markets are the form of economic organization producing the maximum value output in society.

From this understanding of economic behavior, economists derive the primary normative conclusion of the CMP, the *Pareto criterion* (named for Vilfredo Pareto, nineteenth-century Italian economist and mathematician). As an ethical principle, the Pareto criterion mandates that no collective action be taken which reduces the welfare of even one individual in the polity. Collective actions are described as consistent with the Pareto criterion when they enhance the welfare of some in polity, without reducing the welfare of any other person. In other words, if "society" were going to pursue some policy that would make even one member of that society worse off, then under the Pareto criterion that person could veto society's action. Pareto's ethical standard of collective action is the basis for economists' application of descriptions of pure competition and economic "efficiency" as normative standards for the social world. Unfortunately, the economic outcome defined by the efficiency standards of pure competition is rarely achieved in the real world. Therefore, the CMP has not provided a sustainable ethical basis for economists who desire to convince their audiences of the importance of institutions of private property and free market trading to the overall welfare of society.

CRITICISMS OF THE CMP

Let us detail briefly some of the difficulties that the CMP has faced in providing a logical defense of the ethics of political and economic freedom. The CMP, as defined by the methodology of calculus, was attacked empirically at three points in the twentieth century. First was the Market Power, or Monopoly, Argument, which asserts that there should be no significant market power in free market society. Yet, there are significant examples of market power and industrial concentration (i.e., monopoly) in modern economies, especially in the area of government-provided public goods. The potential advantages of large-scale economic organization cannot be explained by the CMP, and economists have to rely on "natural monopoly" arguments which rest on declining cost functions, themselves counter-revolutionary to CMP.

Second, there has been the Macroeconomics Argument of the Keynesian revolution, in which Keynesian theories seek to overturn CMP in reference to the aggregate economy. In the Keynesian view, the economy is not supposed to work as efficiently (to tend toward socially optimum equilibria) on the large scale. Keynesian macroeconomics represents an attack on CMP by arguing that institutional rigidity disrupts macroeconomic performance. Although largely based on ad hoc notions about economic functioning, the Macroeconomics Argument has introduced theories about money, interest rates, saving and investment, and labor unions which serve to undermine economic conclusions about the allocational performance of free markets. In other words, Keynes and his followers, the advocates of the Macroeconomic Argument, think that the free market does not provide an efficient, fair outcome for society.

The third criticism is the Public Goods, or "Market Failure," Argument, which refers to situations where the demand for goods is collective, and property rights are not easily defined. This argument alone seems to justify the need for government regulation of the economy that contradicts the CMP. The Public Goods Argument represents the most legitimate challenge to CMP because it uses rational economic arguments against the primary conclusions about the efficiency of market outcomes. Public goods problems highlight the theoretical difficulties of the CMP in the face of opportunistic behavior, known in Game Theory as "free riding." These arguments reduce the strength of the ethical defense of free markets and social institutions derived from private property arrangements by introducing apparent conflict between economic actions by individuals and the welfare of society in general. Thus the CMP has not provided a convincing moral argument for economic free markets and/or political freedom.

Social Welfare Functions

To handle these criticisms, economists operating within the CMP have turned to the use of *social welfare functions*. Social welfare functions are attempts to objectify society's norms and preferences. In "Rationality and Social Choice," his Presidential Address to the American Economic Association in 1995, game theorist Amartya Sen describes the connection between our ability to make aggregate social welfare judgments and our understanding of social decision-making mechanisms. To Sen, economists must explore the question, Are interest groups rational? In this discussion, we must first determine whether our normative evaluation of political systems will be based on (A) consequences or (B) procedures/rules.

The traditional utilitarian approach to social welfare problems (which are, or must become, consequence-based value judgments) has failed to produce scientific criteria for meaningful ethical evaluation of collective action. Economists' description of society, founded upon social welfare functions and based upon utilitarianism (of the cruder sort, associated with the works of Jeremy Bentham and John Stuart Mill) immediately repudiates the first major principle of modern economic science: that all values are subjective and limited to those who hold them. Because the CMP, like all positivist theories, assumes that all values are subjective, the CMP then fails to account for the objective reality of social norms. The CMP fails to provide a bridge between an ethical relativism of subjective individual values and social norms.

Sen asserts that the analytical tools of Game Theory seek to reconcile the nature of individual economic behavior with concepts of social rationality. In the past, economists have followed the CMP by describing social welfare functions in the attempt to provide an economic model of collective choice (analogous to choice models of neo-classical economic individual rationality) with a normative content. Social welfare functions assign a set of normative values (preferences) to allow economists to proceed towards a cost/benefit analysis of collective actions to determine their "efficiency." This utilitarian model of public interest assumes that government is maximizing "social welfare." The "social choice" school of Nobel Laureate Kenneth Arrow carries mathematical formulation of social welfare functions to the highest mathematical level.

Unfortunately, Arrow's Impossibility Theorem, in which irrelevant alternatives (dominating strategies) are independent of each other, repudiates the entire economic approach to developing a universal social welfare function. Sen's comments indicate that we cannot have a universal social welfare function which would be a Pareto optimal nondictatorship. The player's preferences must include some constitutional values, preferences over rules of the social game itself. Only if we can sum utilities in cardinal calculus and make interpersonal utility comparisons, can we then decide a social welfare function.[1] But this is in direct contradiction to the principle tenets of the CMP. In other words, the CMP with calculus alone does not provide an adequate understanding of social norms, while social welfare functions result in a violation of the scientific approach of the CMP. Sen concludes that an evaluation of social welfare cannot rely entirely on consequence-based utilitarianism, but must rest on a game theoretic analysis in which we define liberties and rights as a subset of social strategies which are permissible, within the set of all possible available strategies. The key to the social game is found in examination of the informational content available to players.

THE EVOLUTIONS OF SOCIAL NORMS

Game Theory allows social scientists to describe the evolution of social norms as well as the ethical principles of freedom and markets based on private property that are still consistent with the economic market theory detailed by the CMP. In the version of economic behavior described by the CMP, predation is portrayed as a rational economic strategy. Game Theory succeeds where the CMP fails because it solves the problem of predation, or "opportunistic behavior," that has been the Achilles heel of the CMP and figures prominently in each of the criticisms of economics mentioned above. The most important social circumstance involving predation is described in the Prisoner's Dilemma, a non-cooperative negative-sum game. In the CMP, because of a seeming divergence between individual and community interests, allowing players economic or political freedom produces a result damaging to the interests of society on the whole.

THE PRISONER'S DILEMMA

In the Prisoner's Dilemma, the interests of two partners are placed in conflict by a force outside themselves. As the story goes, two burglars are arrested by the police for a major theft. The police do not have enough solid evidence to convict the two on the big job, but the criminals do not know this. The police separate the burglars, and then place each in a moral dilemma. Each prisoner is told that the other has already confessed and that the judge will throw the book at the fellow who does not confess his crime. If both hold out and do not confess to the big heist, then the police have only enough evidence to convict them on a minor theft, and each will get only a short sentence; if one prisoner confesses, then he goes free, while the other criminal will get a long sentence; and, if both confess, then both get a medium-length sentence.

The best strategy is this: *each prisoner is better off to confess, no matter what his partner does*. Notice that for each criminal, if his partner confesses, then the other will bear the brunt of the penalty; however, it is also in the criminal's interest to confess even in the event that his partner does not. In short, the individual's self-interest, narrowly conceived, is placed in conflict with his interest as a member of the community (note that "community" refers here to the partnership of the criminals, not to the larger social world in which they operate). The criminal is offered the opportunity to betray his partner to improve his own position. This game provides an opportunity to discuss concepts of rationality and self-interest, but more importantly it presents a *lemma* that cannot be solved by the rational process itself. In order to solve the Prisoner's Dilemma, we must conceptualize a moral schema. Some process of communication and cooperation must evolve between the players that transcends the selfish interest of each player.

In the Prisoner's Dilemma, each player can advance his own interests at the cost of the other. In the CMP, this predatory strategy is dominant, meaning that it is the best move no matter whether the opponent is being cooperative or predatory. If the opponent is being cooperative, then playing the predatory strategy allows the player to get off scot-free; while if the opponent is being predatory, then playing the predatory strategy minimizes the damage done by the opponent's strategy choice. Either way, predation is the rational utility-maximizing strategy, yet following it leads both players into the outcome which is the worst for them together as a collective.[2]

The key, as indicated by Sen, is information; neither player knows what the other player is doing. The pure rationality of the payoff matrix indicates that the predatory strategy is dominant; therefore, if this is the only information which the player considers, he will conclude that the other player will also see predation as the dominant strategy.

In the Prisoner's Dilemma there is a divergence between the interests of the individual player and that of the community of players. From the viewpoint of the CMP, pure rationality compels the individual player to adopt the predatory strategy, in defense of his own interests and at the expense of the other player. The game is negative-sum in nature, since the payoff of the player adopting the predatory strategy increases by a smaller amount than the payoff to the opponent decreases. Still, the logic is there; what is rational for the individual is damaging to the community. While it is better to belong to a group (the partnership of the criminals), for the individual criminal it is more beneficial still to get the benefits of membership in the group while looking out exclusively for his own interests (by confessing to the police). Within the CMP, the interests of the individual per se diverge from the interests of the individual as a member of a cooperative partnership. On the other hand, the Prisoner's Dilemma can easily be extended to problems of predation in large groups and in society as a whole. Even though they would prefer a clean environment, individuals may litter, for example, if the costs of littering are going to be borne by all other members of society.

Social norms emerge from the Prisoner's Dilemma that control predation, thus creating an ethical foundation for the efficiency assertions of competitive free markets flowing from the CMP. In the case of the Public Goods Argument, the fear of unchecked predation is utilized to justify government control over many aspects of economic life. For example, in the collection of taxes to finance collective services and in the regulation of pollution, predatory behavior is frequently cited to undermine the argument that the free market will provide economically optimum and efficient outcomes.

Social Norms as Solutions to Predatory Behavior

As it turns out, predation is not the long-run profit-maximizing strategy. Nor are humans so stupid, narrow, and short-sighted that they cannot perceive the importance of the interests of the community in which they live. Here, Game Theory provides an economic understanding of the importance of socially responsible ethical behavior and explains how the rational self-interests of individual players lead to the evolution of social norms conducive to overcoming the problem of predation through ethics. Game Theory shows that "tit-for-tat," reciprocity, is the ultimate economic strategy and thus how political freedom for all individuals is the ultimate ethical principle.

Social norms emerge from the Prisoner's Dilemma that control predation, thus creating an ethical foundation for the efficiency assertions of competitive free markets flowing from the CMP. This happens because the individual players begin to understand that their own predatory behavior provokes predatory behavior in the opponent, which results in a lower payoff to themselves. The individual player learns that what happens to him depends upon the strategy choices of the other player, which is conditioned by his own strategy choices; if the first player is predatory, then the other player is consistently predatory in retaliation. Players who develop a reputation for cooperation enjoy a decidedly greater long-run payoff than those who become known as predators. Thus in the long run, predatory behavior is not as successful as cooperative behavior, and the interests of the individual and the community coincide.

Notice that Game Theory provides a rational and self-interested argument in favor of cooperation, an economics of ethics, as it were.[3]

SOCIAL INSTITUTIONS AND FREE MARKETS

As discussed previously, the CMP did not provide an adequate theoretical framework for describing the importance of social institutions, such as free markets. Game Theory can bridge this gap by explaining how social institutions emerge from rational economic behavior. Game Theory posits that institutional arrangements evolve as non-formal means for overcoming problems of opportunistic behavior. Institutions represent explicitly the moral content found in solution to the ethical dilemmas inherent in opportunism. Personal morality of trust, loyalty, punctuality, and discipline are given social form in an institutional setting. Without these virtues, the opportunistic temptations would undermine cooperative activities.

Institutions represent the collectivization of morality. In the large numbers settings of mass society, it would not be practical to rely on small-scale interpersonal agreements to reduce opportunism to acceptable levels. Institutions such as firms, political parties, and churches promote economies of scale in the indoctrination of morals by mass groups. They give practical, substantive, and recognizable form to the metamoralities of entrepreneurship, ideology, and religion. Institutions evolve to facilitate social cooperation in instances where direct contracting is not practical (too costly). Firms are networks of contracts, but not necessarily explicit contracts. Institutions, then, are a form of exchange between individuals and are thus fully compatible with the economic description of human nature from the CMP but also consistent with a social ethic of political freedom.

At this point the work of Nobel Laureate Friedrich A. Hayek, particularly his concept of the "spontaneous order," provides the critical link between our Game Theory analysis and the ethical value of political and economic freedom. Hayek emphasizes that the benefits of economic exchange are not limited to the parties directly involved. Further, the central social science observation emerging from economics is that human society evolves institutions to overcome any equilibria of existing relations that are Pareto suboptimal, that is, arrangements in which one person will benefit at the expense of others. Even when players have directly opposite interests, as in the negative-sum game of the Prisoner's Dilemma, they find a way to reach an agreement to minimize their collective damage. As social norms evolve, predatory strategies are replaced by cooperative strategies.

Hayek has explained that as civilization progresses, the institutions of society instill within individuals norms of cooperative behavior (or at least, nonpredatory behavior). The violent predatory strategies of the primitive natural world are gradually modified, ritualized, and socially marginalized, and thus destructive coercive competition is replaced by productive economic competition, fostered and maintained, within social institutions based on ethics of political freedom. Such a society is referred to as a "spontaneous order" (similar to Adam Smith's "invisible hand") because, consistent with Game Theory explanations, knowledge and order, laws and social norms are not created by direct legislative action as with social welfare functions, but rather, emerge from the social process as an evolutionary outcome. Put another way, play of the social game educates players towards ethical norms which increase the well-being and productivity of society. Thus there is a vital relationship between freedom and the evolution of a cooperative spontaneous order. Freedom does not imply predation, greed and criminality, but rather, freedom benefits society because there is no long-run divergence between individual and community interests. Game Theory helps us to understand that individual freedom is necessary for the emergence of social norms and institutions which ultimately promote the well-being of society and all of the individuals in that society.

Game Theory offers a merger of the ethics of free markets which emphasize cooperative economic action and overcomes the main criticism of the CMP, i.e., predatory behavior. Game Theory explains the evolution of cooperative solutions to predatory situations, like those in the Prisoner's Dilemma, as the result of rational self-interested (i.e., economic) behavior. The CMP, with its normative standard of the Pareto criterion and its heretofore inadequate support for free markets and free governments (because it did not provide protection against predatory behavior), is the ethical legacy of Western neo-classical economics. Voluntary social relations, viewed as exchanges and contracts, are mutually beneficial to the players and enhance the welfare of society. These voluntary and mutually beneficial exchanges explain why free market economists like Hayek have always argued that political interference with economic exchange will create inefficiencies that reduce the aggregate wealth and welfare of society. Seen from the perspective of Game Theory, social equilibria become self-enforcing contracts. Any attempt to solve the problem of predation through social welfare functions and the use of coercive governmental programs, which seek to replace human freedom by what amounts to state-sponsored predation, are thus a retreat from true ethical progress. In this case, social equilibria are mutually destructive because they merely force predatory behavior to another level, that of the social institutions themselves.

Hayek has always emphasized that coercive solutions to the problems of predation, as for instance, the Social Contract theory, are the intellectual legacy of the Imperial tradition. Rationality seems to dictate that sometimes it is strategically advantageous to engage in predatory behavior. The flaw in the CMP was that it could not justify the existence of social norms and thus could not explain why predation (opportunism) was not consistent with efficient economic behavior. Economics seemed to demonstrate that predatory behavior was rational and, therefore, that market behavior had no ethical basis.

Game Theory demonstrates that economic behavior does not advocate or condone predatory or anti-social behavior. Rather, according to the economics of Game Theory, the opposite is the case; that is, when individuals' interests are in direct opposition, they still find a way to evolve cooperative solutions that resemble the productive outcomes most similar to those of free markets. Economic behavior does not imply anti-social action. When modified by Game Theory, the economics of the CMP leads to evolution of cooperative social norms which refute the seeming strategic advantages of predation. The free market evokes and promotes an ethical code which is cooperative in nature and thus beneficial to society. In this manner, Game Theory provides the crucial link between economic science and ethics. Through Game Theory we come to understand that while human nature is fundamentally economic, it is also social and thus cooperative; when human beings are allowed to be free, it is in their self-interest to evolve social institutions that minimize predation and maximize social welfare.

CONCLUSION

Another Nobel Laureate, James M. Buchanan, has suggested that Game Theory is the mathematics of human interaction. A full-scale argument on the ethics of free markets and government intervention is beyond the scope of this paper. Here it can only be suggested that, with the institutions of private property, the social significance of voluntary market exchanges, and the tremendous ethical potential for social norms of self-government, freedom is the last word in social justice.

A common perception is that the ethics of business is greed and self-interest unconcerned with any aspect of society's welfare. The Classical Microeconomic Paradigm has failed to provide a convincing defense of the free market, for it does not give a basis for understanding the importance of ethical conduct in business relations. Economic science, sometimes connected to partisan politics, is supposed to be the amoral or immoral argument for every sort of crude materialism, the claim that money is the only thing that matters, etc. Yet, nothing could be further from the truth; for Game Theory shows that economics is fully consistent with ethical conduct.

Certainly, classical microeconomics had grossly underdescribed the importance of social institutions; however, Game Theory provides a way to correct for this defect by demonstrating the relevance of ethics for successful conduct in business. By describing how social norms evolve from the process of human interaction, Game Theory provides a rational and logical justification for the ethics of business—honesty, thrift, dependability, punctuality, courtesy, and service.

The ultimate lesson becomes an understanding of the *a priori* necessity for a system of cooperative norms in order to overcome the temptation of predation which humans experience in the social world. Game Theory offers a highly promising vehicle by which to introduce students to contemplation of the role of social norms, i.e., morals, in business circumstances. Game Theory possesses a wide array of technical concepts for study of ethical behavior. Using Game Theory, students may approach a broad number of topics in economics and business. Perhaps this methodology may contribute to a refinement of the student's understanding of the nature of competition and cooperation and of the importance of a firm ethical foundation in the pursuit of excellence.

NOTES

1. Ordinal utility functions are consistent with the essential theoretical precepts of the CMP. An ordinal utility function specifies the ranking of a person's preferences (i.e., their first choice, their second choice, their third, etc.). Unfortunately, the ordinal utility functions of different persons cannot be directly compared. Social welfare functions must use cardinal utility, where the preferences of persons are not only ranked, but given "point values," which then allow direct calculations of utility across groups of persons. Under this approach, the preferences of society as a whole could be calculated, which would allow economists to determine the efficiency of "social" choice in the same fashion which the CMP evaluates the efficiency of individual choices.
2. The Prisoner's Dilemma is only one of many analytical "games" which are provided by the mathematics of Game Theory. Among other things, various types of games are useful in describing the importance of communications between players, or of the information available to players, the nature and stability of equilibria, and so forth.
3. This argument was first elucidated by Robert Axelrod (1984). Some excellent surveys of basic game theory include Gibbons (1997), Reny (1992), Brandenberger (1992), and Rasmusen (1989). Among others, economists who have carried game theory concepts into the description of social equilibria are Sugdon (1989), Young (1996), and Elster (1989).

QUESTIONS FOR DISCUSSION

1. How does the Pareto criterion, which mandates that no collective action be taken that reduces the welfare of even one individual, match your understanding about individual rights?

2. If you act from a position of considering only consequences, would you still come to understand the value of cooperation?

4. Does game theory shift our interpretation of what it means to survive?

5. Could cooperation come to represent the "fittest" in survival of the fittest thinking? If so, how?

6. How would you want others to choose for you if you could not choose?

7. How does one shift from Classical Microeconomic Paradigm to Game Theory thinking? Why?

8. In what context are Game Theory values important? When and why would you be attracted to Game Theory thinking and action?

9. In choosing partners, why would you select a cooperative partner? Are there times or circumstances in which you would select a predator partner?

KILLING AND ALLOWING TO DIE

L. Alan Sasser

ABSTRACT

There is a constant tension in American culture around the issue of the value of life. Conflict arises in consideration of such disparate matters as abortion, capital punishment, suicide, and the like. Technological advances in this century have exaggerated the conflicts and nowhere more evidently than in the practice of medicine. The capability to impact quality of life through the application of technology is just beginning to be understood by persons across the spectrum of philosophical, theological, psychological, and sociological disciplines. One issue that focuses the conflict and raises serious ethical questions is physician-assisted suicide. This paper addresses the issue and offers a retrospective case analysis defending the ethical treatment of human life as valuable and sacred.

My first critically formative experience with the ethical dynamics involving dying and death occurred on my tenth birthday. I was with my maternal grandparents for the summer. I had hinted that what I most wanted for my present that year was a Daisy Air Rifle. I hopped out of bed on my birthday, and on the coffee table was a package that contained the rifle. After my grandfather left for work, I told my grandmother that I was going to take my gun out into the field behind the house and do some hunting. Her last words to me were, "You be careful."

I loaded the gun's chamber with the tiny copper pellets and headed out the door to the large field. There, I was certain to find "big game." I was not disappointed. Perched on a lower limb of a huge oak tree in the middle of the field was a tiny sparrow. I lifted the rifle to my shoulder, locked the bird in my sight, and squeezed the trigger. Much to my surprise and shock, the bird fell to the ground. Quickly I ran over to the base of the tree. There, on the ground, lay the bird. It was not dead—mortally wounded—but not dead. I knelt on the ground and lifted that tiny bird into my hands. Its eyes looked at me and its breast raised and lowered rapidly, erratically.

Suddenly, I was confronted with a dilemma. I took the bird to the house, holding it in my hand. I found my grandmother and told her my story. She outlined what she saw as my options. I could finish what I had started by simply crushing the bird in my hand. Or I could wait for it to die on its own. I am not sure why, but I chose the latter option. Walking out of the house and back to the oak tree, I sat at the foot of that tree and held that bird in my hands until it died. I remember gently stroking its feathers and trying so very carefully to make it as comfortable as I, at age ten, could. When it finally stopped breathing and all its quivering ceased, I buried it and conducted its funeral service. Then I went back to the house and told my grandmother what I had done. What I did not realize then was that I had made a specific value judgment about life, a judgment to which I have consistently returned.

Forty years have passed since that formative experience, but the issues raised for me around ending the life of that creature continue to pose a significant question. Is there is a moral difference between active and passive euthanasia? My intention is to review some of the relevant conversation about the issue and then present a case analysis in which this ethical issue is prominent.

THE FACETS OF EUTHANASIA

Euthanasia has been variously defined, but the most literal definition of the term is "good or easy death." Don V. Bailey provides a helpful discussion of four terms describing forms of euthanasia: voluntary, passive; voluntary, active; involuntary, passive; and involuntary, active.[1] *"Voluntary, passive euthanasia"* is something on the order of palliative care. Efforts are made to keep persons as comfortable as possible without resorting to unusual measures of intervention on the part of the caregiver(s). The inevitability of death is medically indicated and recognized by clinicians as well as by the patients themselves. Efforts are undertaken to ensure patient autonomy and best interest. The patient is aware of and participates in the decision-making.

In the case of *"voluntary, active euthanasia,"* the care-giver(s) plays a more active role in hastening the death of the patient. This may take the form of withdrawal of artificial or mechanical life support apparatus, the intensification of pharmacotherapies, and/or assisted suicide.

"Involuntary, passive euthanasia" recognizes that the patient is not involved in decision-making regarding treatment. Perhaps the patient is incapable of participation for a variety of reasons; other responsible parties do not intervene either to hasten death or prolong life.

Finally, *"involuntary, active euthanasia"* may be described as the intervention by a second or third party in decision-making about a patient's continued life or hastened death without consultation with the patient or the primary caregiver(s).

THE CONVERSATION AMONG ETHICISTS

I can imagine a situation in which I might be asked by a family member, a close friend, or someone with whom I have had a long and endearing relationship to be an accomplice in the hastening of that person's death. At this point the issue of the moral distinction between active and passive euthanasia is enjoined. And on this issue, ethicists are not of one accord. James Rachels has argued that there is not a sufficiently important moral distinction between killing someone who is terminally ill and allowing that same person to die.[2] Tom Beauchamp and James Childress offer a compelling argument for maintaining the distinction.[3] In "Foregoing Life-Sustaining Food and Water: Is It Killing?"[4] Dan W. Brock, M.D., argues persuasively that there is no peculiar moral distinction between killing and allowing to die. Helene A. Lutz' "Ethical Perspectives on the Right to Die: A Case Study," sets forth the complexities of the issue.[5] As Beauchamp and Childress, in another work, state:

> We have also seen that the language of killing is so confusing—causally, legally, and morally—that we should avoid it in discussions of euthanasia and assistance in dying. It is often morally and conceptually more satisfactory to discuss these issues exclusively in the language of optional and obligatory treatments, dispensing altogether with *killing* and *letting die.*[6]

While it may be arguable that a moral distinction between killing and allowing to die is irrelevant when considering an individual situation or a particular case, it is a matter of profound significance when one is considering social or public policy that will eventually find itself expressed in the legal corpus and thereby become the law of the land. Even Dr. Brock, at the conclusion of the article cited above, states: "Moreover, sound public policy should reflect additional considerations, such as slippery-slope worries about abuse."[7]

In "Deciding for Yourself: The Objections," Daniel Maguire makes a provocative observation: "It is fair to say that if you do not know the objections to your position, you do not know your position."[8] He elucidates the arguments used to reject active euthanasia and shows their fallacies. The one argument he fails to address is what the potentially routine involvement of physicians in carrying out the wishes of terminally ill patients to end their lives would do to alter the public perception of health care providers. Interestingly, Beauchamp and Childress do address this issue in the Fourth Edition of their *Principles of Biomedical Ethics*:

> Physicians have traditionally maintained that they have no obligation to assist in suicide, only an obligation to care for patients in the process of their dying and an obligation to "do no harm." This position suggests that the act of assisting, if justifiable, is never obligatory; at best, it is a merciful form of nonrequired assistance. This attitude needs to change in medicine. We need to reconceive certain forms of assisting in dying as part of the responsibility of caring for the patient, while rejecting other forms of assistance as outside that obligation. The focus of the discussion about euthanasia and assisted suicide in upcoming years should be on traditional attitudes in medicine, the policies they have generated, and ways to redraw the unstable and often indefensible lines in these policies. As these policies are reconsidered for competent patients, we will also need to reconsider policies for incompetent patients.[9]

Back to the question: Is there a distinctive moral difference between killing a patient suffering from a terminal illness, irreversible in its outcome, absolutely certain to bring death, and allowing that same patient to die? Ethicists position themselves at contrasting points and presently there is no unanimity of opinion.

THE CONVERSATION AMONG PHYSICIANS

Physicians and other caregivers are not of one voice either. Gregory E. Pence reflects on one now famous case, the "Debbie" case. He notes the controversy immediately following publication of the letter, "It's Over Debbie," alleged to have been written by an anonymous medical resident, referring to his active euthanasia treatment of a patient who summoned him in the early hours of the morning. Pence observes that four physicians known for their interest in medical ethics wrote a letter in response to the "Debbie" case.

They invoked the example of mercy-killing by physicians in Holland and argued:

> We must say to each of our fellow physicians that we will not tolerate killing of patients and that we shall take disciplinary action against doctors who kill. And we must say to the broader community that if it insists on tolerating or legalizing active euthanasia, it will have to find non-physicians to do the killing.[10]

However, as Pence notes further, one year later, the *New England Journal of Medicine* published a special article by twelve physicians who advocated the opposite position. Many of these physicians, leaders in medical ethics, believed that it was "not immoral" for physicians to assist in the suicide of "hopelessly ill" terminal patients.

Significantly, even in the Netherlands, where decriminalization of mercy killing has been given wide acceptance, Dutch physicians are still divided in their attitudes, practices, and experience. The "slippery slope" argument employed by ethicists as a metaphor for the potentially far-reaching consequences of actions or practices is regularly employed in discussions of physician-assisted suicide or involuntary, active euthanasia.[11]

WHEN DYING BEGINS

Let me approach this from another angle. Dying begins from the very moment of conception, whether in a mother's womb or a laboratory petri dish. Dying and death are, therefore, parts of life, not to be looked upon as alien intruders but as the culmination of human existence and experience.

From this premise, we certainly seek to protect, sustain, and preserve life. We also recognize that people die and that there are limits for sustenance and preservation. Our recognition of these limits does not formulate the grounds for an active, intentional hastening of death; however, such recognition of limits can, and very often does, create a context in which passive euthanasia may be the inevitable outcome.

An ethical exploration of these issues is essential, especially when it forms part of the experience of those facing their own dying as well as those providing for their care in the process. An ethics of care such as that articulated by Carol Gilligan[12] and others, as well as an ethics of virtue, expressed in the writings of Aristotle, Anselm, and most recently Alasdair MacIntyre,[13] wedded to consideration of ethical principles like autonomy, beneficence, nonmaleficence, justice, and proportionality are indispensable components of a deliberative process that seeks to address this issue.

When Claude Thompson, professor of systematic theology in the Candler School of Theology of Emory University, was in his sixties, he learned he had a malignancy. As he meditated about his condition, he expressed these ideas to God: (1) that he could die; (2) that he could happily experience divine healing; (3) that he could live under a handicap. However, he told God the one thing he was unwilling to do was to endure his illness alone, on his own strength.

Just as Thompson did not want to die alone, any discussion of allowing someone who is in the final stages of life to die must be accompanied by a commitment from appropriate care-givers to be there at the end. The decision to forego medical treatment, once it has been arrived at and through whatever means are employed, must also be accompanied by a commitment to attend to the care of the dying person with comfort and love and physical presence, but never abandonment.

As Carol Gilligan says, "Attachment and separation anchor the cycle of human life, describing the biology of human reproduction and the psychology of human development."[14] Among the many things this means, certainly, is that the way we care for our dying reveals something very meaningful about the ultimate value we place on human life. Therefore, at the very least, until our culture is willing and able to extend to every human being the highest and best level of medical care and treatment, then we must not allow the moral distinction between active euthanasia and passive euthanasia to vanish. For with its disappearance, the connectedness that unites us and binds us in a common humanity also vanishes.

BACKGROUND TO A CASE STUDY

GH (initials are used to protect confidentiality) is a 73-year-old male suffering from herpes zoster, the medical term for shingles. Herpes zoster is an infection of the nerves that supply certain areas of the skin. It causes a painful rash of crusting blisters that can cover extensive portions of the face and torso. In cases in which the face is affected, it can cause blindness. The physician who initially diagnosed GH and the several specialists who have treated him have told him that his is the most severe case they have ever seen. The rash covers his body from the lower part of his ribs up beyond his neck and onto his face. Although he is not yet blind, his physicians expect that he will lose sight in the near future. There is no cure for his illness, and his quality of life will deteriorate as he gets older.

By the end of 1991, after months of careful thought, GH decided that he could not take the pain any longer and that he wanted to end his life. Because of his own discomfort with violence and his fear that his attempt might be unsuccessful, as well as a genuine concern for any family members who might find his body, he decided that suicide by lethal dose of medication was the avenue for him.

To improve his efforts at persuasion, GH did some research in bioethics literature and found Joseph Fletcher's defense of both assisted suicide and active euthanasia. Writing in "Ethics and Euthanasia," Dr. Fletcher says,

> It is harder morally to justify letting somebody die a slow and ugly death, dehumanized, than it is to justify helping him escape from such misery...The case for euthanasia depends upon how we understand "benefit of the sick" and "harm" and "wrong." If we regard dehumanized and merely biological life as sometimes real harm and the opposite of benefit, to refuse to welcome or even introduce death would be quite wrong morally.[15]

Despite the power of Fletcher's arguments and his persistent pleas for help, GH was unable to convince his physicians to help him. He opted instead to search for a physician who might be willing to help him.

ANALYSIS OF THE CASE

There are several ways to do bioethical case analysis. One method that combines the work of several theorists is called the Four-Step Method for Retrospective Case Analysis. This approach to case analysis has been popularized by ethicists and clinicians affiliated with the University of Virginia School of Medicine. The process looks at cases after the fact, hence the retrospective feature. Included in the methodology are the following:

Step 1:   Assemble Relevant Facts
A.   Medical facts and indications for treatment
B.   Patient preferences and quality of life
C.   Contextual factors and legal concerns

Step 2:   Identify Ethical Problem(s)
A.   Identify, describe, and rank ethical problem(s)
B.   Search for analogous cases

Step 3:   Identify Ethical Guidelines for Clinicians
A.   Summarize existing guidelines/recommendations

Step 4:   Engage in Dialogue and Resolution
A.   List options
B.   Evaluate options and conflicting claims
C.   Rank options and decide, giving reasons

Using this four-step process, the following is an analysis of GH's case.

GH is a 73-year-old male, intelligent enough to do research in bioethics literature. He lives at home with his wife. There are other family and perhaps extended family. It is likely that, because of his age at the time of his diagnosis, insurance coverage is supplemented by Medicare. His family is reported to be extremely supportive and actively involved in his care. He is from a strong religious heritage that decries suicide as punishable by eternal condemnation, a pertinent factor in regard to his expressed desire to have his life ended by unnatural means.

GH has a diagnosis of herpes zoster, commonly known as shingles. It has been an increasingly painful and debilitating disease for him. His treatment has focused on relief of symptoms, as there is no cure for the illness. Though his prognosis is not terminal, the probability is that he will continue to experience increasing pain and debilitation and a steadily eroding quality of life. Recommendations for continuing treatment include additional medication for pain.

This patient is capable of decision-making and is well informed about his illness. He understands the nature and extent of his disease as he has been living with it for several years. He describes his quality of life as "more pain…than I can handle." His current wish is for lethal administration of drugs to end his life (i.e., physician-assisted suicide). Regarding preferences of family/surrogate decision makers, GH's family members have been "extremely supportive and actively involved in his care" and they "would be strongly opposed to his plans to commit suicide."

GH has experienced intense suffering and pain in spite of a host of pharmacotherapies as well as surgical interventions, so much so that his weight is down to 94 pounds from what would have been a baseline of 150 pounds. There is little question about the patient's preference. He has made clear his desire to have his life terminated, at least to his physicians; it is not entirely clear whether his spouse or family members know the intensity of his wish.

The resources and strategies for helping this patient cope involve continued interaction with medical caregivers as well as supportive interaction with his family, all of which appear available to the patient.

Apparent institutional factors in this case include the fact that, according to *The American College of Physicians Ethics Manual*, mercy killing, assisted suicide, and euthanasia remain prohibited by law in the United States. In point of fact, seven states have decriminalized physician-assisted suicide and even highly public figures such as Dr. Jack Kevorkian have not been successfully prosecuted in the 43 states where physician-assisted suicide is banned by law.[16] Moreover, there is an apparent conflict between clinicians who have been treating this patient and who have consistently refused to be compliant in his death wish and a physician in a neighboring community who has indicated a willingness to comply in the patient's wish.

Ethical considerations include a conflict of principles. The patient's autonomy is contrasted with his physicians' adherence to the principles of beneficence and non-malevolence. The most obvious legal consideration is that physician-assisted suicide remains against the law. Ethical guidelines and standards uniformly support physicians acting so as to save and enhance the lives of patients rather than to terminate them. What, then, are the ethically acceptable options?

With regard to this patient, refusal to comply with his request for a physician-assisted suicide is the only acceptable ethical option. If GH were suffering from a terminal disease with an irreversible and imminent mortality, there might be cause for consideration of an alternate course of treatment. Beauchamp and Childress have argued that

> [M]erciful physician interventions in the form of voluntary active euthanasia are not inherently wrong or incompatible with the role of a health professional. Nonetheless, public policies that sanction such physician activities are unacceptable unless they are accompanied by extraordinarily careful regulation and monitoring. Second, we argue that prohibitions in biomedical ethics against certain forms of assisted suicide should be eased, making physicians more comfortable in helping certain patients achieve what for them is a comfortable and timely death.[17]

Such is not the case, however, with this patient. With regard to the apparent dispute between the clinicians consulted in this case, appropriate conversation and confrontation regarding pertinent legal realities as well as the ethical considerations arising from medicine's historic and contemporary role in society certainly are in order. In addition, consultation on additional medically indicated treatment to reduce or relieve further pain/suffering for the patient is in order. The obvious conflict presented here has its origin in the patient's right to autonomy, including death, which runs headlong into the legal, social, and professional codes that forbid killing.

Justification given for the preferred resolution of this case is that the patient's right to self-determination, his autonomy—including the right to refuse treatment—is not absolute. It does not, in practice, extend to the free choice of death in lieu of prolonged suffering and loss of dignity. The rights of this patient at this juncture conflict with prevailing laws, accepted social mores, and codes of ethics in medicine, including the Hippocratic oath, which seek to protect persons from harm. Again, however, in this instance, the patient in question is not suffering from a terminal illness, however debilitating his actual disease may be; and were his condition terminal, then the nature of his treatment might differ.

The American Medical Association, Council on Ethical and Judicial Affairs sets forth the organization's position regarding ethical and legal limits on the physician's agency in a patient's death:

> Although a patient may refuse a medical intervention and the physician may comply with this refusal, the physician must never intentionally and directly cause death or assist a person to commit suicide.[18]

Satisfactory resolution of this case will ultimately necessitate involvement of clinicians who have differing opinions of physician-assisted suicide in conversation with one another as well as inclusion in such conversation of the patient and patient's family.

In terms of the ongoing care of this patient, renewed and perhaps more aggressive therapeutic intervention by his primary physicians is one possible indication. Moreover, as indicated above, the involvement of the patient, his family, and other appropriate caregivers in providing the highest level and quality of comfort care for this patient is of paramount significance.

Although Dr. D. has stated that he has every intention of complying with the patient's wish for a physician-assisted suicide, his reluctance to act arbitrarily and unilaterally indicates some reservation as well as some desire to test what repercussions there might be from his actions, both legally and professionally.

CONCLUSION

This essay began with a true story of an early personal ethical dilemma. In that instance, my own action created the dilemma. The sparrow did not come to me seeking an end to its life. I occasioned its death by my personal actions in mortally wounding it with an air rifle. As I understand it, simply crushing that bird in my hands would have been voluntary, active euthanasia. My action on that occasion was involuntary, passive euthanasia. Would it have taken more courage for the former than the latter? I do not know. I do know that birds and human beings do not have the same capacity for participation in the kinds of decision-making faced by patients, physicians, ethicists, and other clinicians in the increasingly complex environment of tertiary care medicine.

This discipline of biomedical or clinical ethics is still in its formative years. The introduction and prevalent use of technologies unheard of a generation ago has revolutionized medical practice in this country and around the world. The development of ethics committees or ethics consult services in tertiary care settings such as hospitals and skilled care nursing facilities are one evidence of the increased demand for careful and sensitive consideration of patient treatment and medical practice. As the case of GH and its analysis have demonstrated, questions of appropriate clinical intervention, responsiveness of caregivers to patients, conflicts arising out of competing ethical principles, and the diverse nature of public apprehension about all these issues are undergoing considerable transition. Perhaps the absence of any single or unquestioned authoritative moral tradition in our pluralistic society, coupled with the complexity of our nation's delivery of health care, makes such conflict inevitable. At the very least, it mandates continued conversation and informed deliberation about the right thing to do.

NOTES

1. Don V. Bailey, *The Challenge of Euthanasia* (Lanham, MD: University Press of America, 1990), 33-39.
2. James Rachels, "Active and Passive Euthanasia," in *Ethical Issues in Death and Dying*, ed. Robert F. Weir (New York: Columbia University Press, 1986), 249-256.
3. Tom Beauchamp and James Childress, "Killing and Letting Die," in *Ethical Issues in Death and Dying*, 257-266.
4. Dan W. Brock, "Foregoing Life-Sustaining Food and Water: Is It Killing?" in *By No Extraordinary Means*, ed. Joanne Lynn (Indianapolis: Indiana University Press, 1986), 117-131.
5. Helene A. Lutz, "Ethical Perspectives on the Right to Die: A Case Study," in *To Die or Not to Die*, eds. Arthur S. Berger and Joyce Berger (New York: Praeger Publishers, 1990), 25-39.
6. Tom Beauchamp and James Childress, *Principles of Biomedical Ethics*, 4th ed. (New York: Oxford University Press, 1994), 225.
7. Brock, 131.
8. Daniel Maguire, "Deciding for Yourself: The Objections," *Ethical Issues in Death and Dying*, 284.
9. Beauchamp and Childress, *Principles of Biomedical Ethics*, 241.
10. Gregory E. Pence, *Classic Cases in Medical Ethics* (New York: McGraw-Hill Publishing Company, 1990), 45-46.
11. The so-called "slippery slope" is a metaphor in ethical and political conversation. It refers to the image of an issue or a situation that depicts society perched on the edge of a cliff or steep slope. Moral principles are something like the guardrail which prevents falling. The idea is that if enough of the moral guards are removed, a falling will occur, the end result of which will be detrimental to the entire well-being of the society.
12. Carol Gilligan, *In a Different Voice* (Cambridge, MA: Harvard University Press, 1982).
13. Alasdair MacIntyre, *Three Rival Versions of Moral Enquiry: Encyclopedia, Genealogy, and Tradition* (Notre Dame, IN: University of Notre Dame Press, 1990).
14. Gilligan, 151.
15. Joseph Fletcher, "Ethics and Euthanasia," in *To Live and to Die*, ed. Robert H. Williams (New York: Springer-Verlag, 1973), 113-122.
16. Lori Montgomery, "Doctors Begin Talking of Suicide Standards," *Raleigh (NC) News & Observer*, 27 September 1996.
17. Beauchamp and Childress, *Principles of Biomedical Ethics*, 227.
18. "Report 12: Euthanasia," *The American Medical Association, Council on Ethical and Judicial Affairs* (Chicago: American Medical Association, 1986), Sections 2:18 and 2:19.

QUESTIONS FOR DISCUSSION

1. What role does pain management play in this discussion of patient comfort and assisted suicide?

2. Would a tolerance of, or legalization of, mercy killing damage our cultural values?

3. At what point is life no longer worth living? Who can decide this and how?

4. When do we learn to be caregivers? How can we make a difference at the end of a person's life in effective and nurturing ways? What constitutes this level of commitment?

5. People disagree over the phrase "highest and best level of medical care." Why do you think the term is so controversial? What does it mean to you?

6. How do we know what the right thing to do is? In the case study presented in this article, is the decision to do the right thing solely based on the law against physicians practicing assisted suicide?

7. Does prolonged suffering necessarily result in loss of dignity?

CONTRIBUTORS

REBECCA F. BLOMGREN has been a member of the Greensboro College faculty since 1988. She is the Director of the College's Teacher Education Program and Professor of Education. She has served as an editor of several education texts and authored articles on critical theory in education.

JUDY BLANKENSHIP CHEATHAM is Professor of English and Campbell Chair of Writing at Greensboro College. Her teaching and research interests include adult literacy, American literature, and women's studies.

GEORGE CHEATHAM is Professor of English at Greensboro College. In addition to introductory English courses, his teaching and research interests include Renaissance literature and 20th-century British and American literature.

RICHARD FRANCIS CRANE is Assistant Professor of History at Greensboro College. He is the author of a book on the French army and foreign policy between the world wars, and he is presently working on a study of British appeasement in the late 1930s.

CHARLES HEBERT is Associate Professor of English at Greensboro College. He teaches early American and world literature in addition to first-year composition, journalism, creative writing, and business and administrative writing.

JOHN HEMPHILL is Associate Professor of Education at Greensboro College. He is building a database of proverbial wisdom from a variety of cultures and sources, and he is in the process of compiling the proverbs into a book of cross-cultural wisdom.

DANIEL N. KECK is Vice President for Academic Affairs and Dean of the Faculty at Greensboro College. He also has an appointment as Professor of Political Science. He has held faculty and senior-level administrative positions at Baldwin-Wallace College, Carthage College, and Lindenwood College. He is a member of the Board of Directors of the Triad World Affairs Council.

THOMAS A. LANGFORD served as Chair of the Department of Religion and Dean of the Divinity School, and he is now Provost Emeritus of Duke University. His primary fields of study have been philosophical theology and Methodist theology.

RAY MARTIN is Associate Professor of Art and Art Education at Greensboro College. His paintings have been exhibited in numerous one-man and group shows. He has collaborated with musicians, choreographers, theatrical artists and his six-year-old son Vincent in recent years. Selected as an outstanding alumnus of the first twenty-five years of the East Carolina University School of Art, he understands the teaching of art as a spiritual vocation.

CHARLES S. MCCOY is Robert Gordon Sproul Professor Emeritus of Theological Ethics, Pacific School of Religion and Graduate Theological Union, Berkeley, California. He initiated discussions that led to the formation of the Graduate Theological Union and founded the Center for Ethics and Social Policy in Berkeley and the Trinity Center for Ethics and Corporations in New York. Among his many publications are *When gods Change*; *Management of Values*; and *Fountainhead of Federalism*.

NANCY M. MCELVEEN is Professor of French at Greensboro College. She is the author of several articles and reviews on seventeenth-century French topics in various professional journals.

FREDERICK J. OERTHER III, Associate Professor of Economics at Greensboro College, has published several reviews and articles in professional economic journals and has made numerous presentations to regional and international meetings of economists. In addition to Game Theory, his research interests focus on various libertarian and free market concerns.

PHILIP A. ROLNICK is Associate Professor of Religion at Greensboro College. He is the Director of the Ethics Across the Curriculum Program at Greensboro College and the author of *Analogical Possibilities: How Words Refer to God*. His research is equally focused on issues in theology and ethics.

L. ALAN SASSER is Executive Assistant to the President at Greensboro College. He has also served as Dean of the Chapel and Minister to the College, and he has contributed to the academic areas of ethical studies. His post-doctoral studies have concentrated in the field of clinical bioethics, and he has served on hospital ethics consult services.

W. BARNES TATUM is Professor of Religion and Philosophy at Greensboro College. His teaching and research interests lie in the area of Biblical literature and Christian origins, especially the Gospels and Jesus. His monographs include *In Quest of Jesus: A Guidebook* (1982); *John the Baptist and Jesus: A Report of the Jesus Seminar* (1994); and *Jesus at the Movies: A Guide to the First Hundred Years* (1997). A member of the American Academy of Religion and the Society of Biblical Literature, he has published articles and reviews in various professional journals.

JEFFREY WATTLES teaches philosophy at Kent State University. He is the author of *The Golden Rule* (Oxford University Press, 1996) and is currently working on a manuscript on the philosophy of living. Wattles has been a North Carolina Visiting Scholar, Greensboro College's Jean Fortner Ward Lecturer, and the recipient of grants from the John Templeton Foundation and the Ohio Humanities Council.

CRAVEN E. WILLIAMS is the seventeenth President of Greensboro College. He has previously served as President of Gardner-Webb University and Vice President of Davidson College and Mary Baldwin College, where he taught religion and psychology. A regular contributor to educational and religious publications, Dr. Williams is the author of *A Wesley Primer*, an introduction to the lives and work of John and Charles Wesley.